Healthy Teens

SUCCESS IN HIGH SCHOOL
AND BEYOND

Dedication

For my five children, Wally, David, Sharon, Jim, and Bill.
You are grown up now and I am proud of you.
Your support for my work has made a significant difference.

Healthy Teens

SUCCESS IN HIGH SCHOOL AND BEYOND

SECOND EDITION

ALICE R. McCARTHY, PH.D.

Bridge Communications, Inc.
Birmingham, Michigan

Healthy Teens: Success in High School and Beyond was written in part with development funds provided by the Lansing School District, Lansing, Michigan, and the Monroe County Intermediate School District, Monroe, Michigan, through the Monroe/Lenawee Consortium of Drug-Free Schools. The publisher expresses thanks for this assistance.

The idea for the book came from *Tuning In to Twenty-First Century Schools and Teens*, a parent handbook developed for the Wayne County Regional Educational Service Agency in Wayne, Michigan, in 1995. That project was funded by the Children's Trust Fund of Michigan.

Copyright © 1997 by Alice R. McCarthy, Ph.D., and Bridge Communications, Inc.

ISBN 0-9621645-4-2

James H. McCarthy, Writer/Editor
Marcia Rayner Applegate, Associate Writer/Editor
David N. McCarthy, Editor
Book layout/design by Creative Business Services, Warren, Michigan
Cover layout/design by Laura Linenfelser, P.S. Abrams, Inc., Troy, Michigan
Cover photography by Joe Crachiola

Includes annotated resource list.

Printed in the United States of America 1997.

Second Edition
10 9 8 7 6 5 4 3 2 1

Published and distributed by

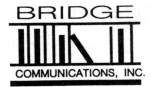

BRIDGE
COMMUNICATIONS, INC.

Books from Bridge Communications, Inc., are available at quantity discounts for educational use. For more information, write to Bridge Communications, Inc., 1450 Pilgrim Road, Birmingham, Michigan 48009, call 810-646-1020, fax 810-644-8546, or e-mail BridgeComm@aol.com. Web site: http://bridge-comm.com. Please write with your comments about *Healthy Teens: Success in High School and Beyond*. Thank you.

Contents

Comprehensive School Health in Michigan

Beginning in 1984, several key state agencies came together in a cooperative effort to improve the health and safety of Michigan's school children and their families. The result of that collaboration was the *Michigan Model for Comprehensive School Health Education.* This nationally recognized school health effort more efficiently uses existing resources, avoids duplication of services, and provides a clear message of disease prevention and health promotion. The *Michigan Model* was developed in cooperation with voluntary and professional organizations, community and parent groups, and private industry, and is being voluntarily used in 93 percent of Michigan public school districts and in more than 200 private schools.

A key element to the success of the *Michigan Model* has been the active involvement of parents as partners in the school health education process. At every level, the *Michigan Model* offers resources and activities that inform parents and involve families. Whether developed with state funds or incorporated from the private sector, these *Good For You!* family education materials suggest resources and activities that will help the family deal with the difficult and disturbing risks that young people face in our society.

The latest resource in this commitment to parents and family involvement is *Healthy Teens: Success in High School and Beyond*, a guide for parents of high school students. Alice R. McCarthy, Ph.D., a nationally recognized author of parent education materials, developed this guide with the input of families, educators, health experts, crime prevention and crisis intervention professionals, and police officers. I hope that you will find this information useful in your efforts to raise healthy, happy teens in these challenging times.

Jean Chabut, Chairperson
Michigan Model State Steering Committee

vii

Acknowledgments

This book was made possible through the efforts of many people. Those listed below provided assistance, resources, knowledge, and skills in contributing to and reviewing the text to ensure that the information provided is accurate. The publisher is deeply grateful for the assistance of so many professionals who care about the health and welfare of adolescents.

Allen Park Parent Volunteers, Joyce Bertasio and Carol Sizemore, Allen Park, Michigan.

Jerry Aris, M.B.A., President, Citizens Against Crime, Allen, Texas.

Patsy Baker, Program Analyst, Rape Prevention and Services Program, Child & Family Services, Michigan Family Independence Agency, Lansing, Michigan.

Laurie Bechhofer, M.P.H., Evaluation Consultant, Supervisor, Comprehensive Programs in Health & Childhood, Michigan Department of Education, Lansing, Michigan.

Michael J. Bender, Principal, and the families of Allen Park High School, Allen Park, Michigan.

Joyce Buchanan, Administrative Assistant to Dr. Lloyd D. Johnston, The University of Michigan *Monitoring the Future* Study, Survey Research Center, Ann Arbor, Michigan.

Jean Chabut, M.P.H., Chief, Center for Health Promotion and Chronic Disease Prevention, Michigan Department of Community Health, Lansing, Michigan.

Jan Christensen, J.D., M.S.W., Chief, Division of Violence, Injury, and Surveillance, Center for Health Promotion and Chronic Disease Prevention, Community Public Health Agency, Lansing, Michigan.

Sue Coats, M.S.W., Program Director, Turning Point, Mt. Clemens, Michigan.

Laura Coens, Director of Communications, Michigan Dyslexia Institute/ Dyslexia Association of America.

Willard R. Daggett, Ed.D., International Center for Leadership in Education, Inc., Schenectady, New York.

Steven W. Enoch, Ed.D., former Superintendent of Schools, Bonsall Union School District in southern California.

Pam Farlow-Wolgast, M.A., L.L.P., L.P.C., C.S.W., Staff Training and Development Coordinator, Common Ground, Pontiac, Michigan.

Holly Fechner, J.D., Labor and Employment Attorney, Policy Office of the U.S. Department of Labor, Takoma Park, Maryland.

Kathy Gibson, School Health Consultant, Center for School Community Outreach, Wayne County Regional Educational Services Agency, Wayne, Michigan.

Althea Grant, M.S.W., A.C.S.W., Executive Director, Detroit Rape Crisis Center, Detroit Receiving Hospital, Detroit, Michigan.

Naomi Haines Griffith, M.A., M.S.W., Executive Director, Parents and Children Together (PACT), Consultant, Alabama Children's Trust Fund, Decatur, Alabama.

Detective Ronald Halcrow, Birmingham Police Department, Birmingham, Michigan.

Ellen Hayse, M.S., Resource Coordinator, Resource Center on Sexual and Domestic Violence, Lansing, Michigan.

John Howell, Ph.D., F/A.O.G.P.E., Director of Abrams Teaching Laboratory and Research, Michigan Dyslexia Institute/Dyslexia Association of America.

Kay Howell, M.A., F/A.O.G.P.E., Michigan Dyslexia Institute/Dyslexia Association of America.

Auleen Jarrett, R.N., B.S.N., President, CRIMEFREE Seminars, Inc., Livonia, Michigan.

Rachel N. Kay, M.P.H., Cook County Department of Public Health, Oak Park, Illinois.

Gloria Krys, M.A., C.S.W., L.P.C., Program Coordinator, Assault Crisis Center of Washtenaw County Community Mental Health, Ypsilanti, Michigan.

Joseph Malgeri, M.S.M., Career Solutions, Troy, Michigan.

The Michigan Department of State Police: Sergeant Joseph Hanley, Special Operations, Traffic Services Division; Lt. Dan Smith, Traffic Services Division; Sergeant Darwin A. Scott, Criminal Intelligence Unit, and Phyllis Good, Supervisor, Narcotics and Dangerous Drugs Unit, East Lansing Laboratory, East Lansing, Michigan.

Katherine Miller, M.A., Prevention Section Chief, Office of Substance Abuse Services, Michigan Department of Community Health, Lansing, Michigan.

Helene Mills, Ed.D., Principal, Seaholm High School, Birmingham, Michigan.

James Moore, Program Director and Assistant Executive Director, American Lung Association, Lansing, Michigan.

Patricia Morgan, R.N., M.S., Consultant for School Health Programs, School Health Unit, Michigan Department of Community Health, Lansing, Michigan.

William T. Munsell, Director of Financial Aid, Lake Superior State University, Sault Sainte, Marie, Michigan.

Sherry Murphy, M.A., Consultant for Drug Free Schools, Oakland Schools Intermediate School District, Waterford, Michigan.

Patricia Nichols, M.S., C.H.E.S., Supervisor, Comprehensive Programs in Health & Early Childhood, Michigan Department of Education, Lansing, Michigan.

Carol Noël, Author, Communications Specialist, President, Serious Business, Inc., Petoskey, Michigan.

Karen Petersmarck, M.P.H., Ph.D., Consultant, Division of Violence, Injury, and Surveillance, Center for Health Promotion and Chronic Disease Prevention, Community Public Health Agency, Lansing, Michigan.

Andrea Poniers, M.S.S.W., Public Health Consultant, Tobacco Section, Center for Health Promotion, Chronic Disease Prevention, Michigan Department of Community Health, Lansing, Michigan.

Randall S. Pope, Chief, HIV/AIDS Prevention & Intervention, Michigan Department of Community Health, Lansing, Michigan.

Lt. Mike Radzik, Washtenaw County Sheriff's Department, Ypsilanti, Michigan.

David Rosen, M.D., M.P.H., C.S. Mott Children's Hospital, A. Alfred Taubman Health Care Center, Ann Arbor, Michigan.

Eli Saltz, Ph.D., Director, The Merrill-Palmer Institute, Detroit, Michigan.

Joy Schumacher, R.N., B.S.N., Oakland County Health Department AIDS Office, Pontiac, Michigan.

Patricia Smith, M.S., Division of Violence, Injury, and Surveillance, Center for Health Promotion and Chronic Disease Prevention, Community Public Health Agency, Lansing, Michigan.

Craig C. Spangler, D.D.S., Bloomfield Hills, Michigan.

Stephen Spector, Ph.D., Psychologist, Beacon Hill Clinic, Birmingham, Michigan.

Lou Stewart, M.A.T., L.D., diagnostician and educational therapist, Birmingham, Michigan.

James Stone, Guidance Counseling Department Head, Groves High School, Birmingham, Michigan.

Donald B. Sweeney, M.A., Chief, School Health Unit, Michigan Department of Community Health, Lansing, Michigan.

Betty Tableman, M.P.A., Director, Prevention Services, Michigan Department of Community Health, Lansing, Michigan.

Lois Thieleke, M.S., Extension Home Economist, Michigan State University Extension, Oakland County, Michigan.

Diane Trippett, M.S., R.D., Clinical Nutrition Manager, Dietetics Department, Children's Hospital of Michigan, Detroit, Michigan.

Waterford Township Police Department, Detective Sergeants Larry Ivory and Michael Oliver, Waterford, Michigan.

Howell Wechsler, Ed.D., M.P.H., Health Scientist, Division of Adolescent Health, Centers for Disease Control and Prevention, Atlanta, Georgia.

Sis Wenger, M.A., Executive Director, National Association for Children of Alcoholics (NACoA), Rockville, Maryland.

Delores Wilson, Counselor, Allen Park Schools, Allen Park, Michigan.

James Windell, M.A., L.L.P., Oakland Psychological Clinic, Oakland County Probate Court, Pontiac, Michigan.

Joel L. Young, M.D., Medical Director, Psychiatric Evaluation and Referral Center, Crittenton Hospital, Rochester, Michigan.

* * * *

The Baldwin Library, Adult Reference Desk, Birmingham, Michigan.

Borders Book Shop, Southfield, Michigan.

Walsh College Library, Walsh College of Accountancy and Business Administration, Troy, Michigan.

Introduction

Adolescence is a time of exploration and discovery—a crucial opportunity for developing the knowledge and practices that make up a healthy life. It is also the time when teens may encounter serious risks to their physical and mental health. Families, schools, and communities have an obligation to provide teens with information about healthy practices and health risks, and to foster the skills and motivation for avoiding risks. Through curriculum, school policy, and clear examples of health-promoting behavior, we can encourage teens to form good health habits and help them recognize that education and health are mutually reinforcing.

Healthy Teens was written to meet three important goals: First, to provide families of adolescent children with a single, authoritative, and easy-to-use reference about the most important health, developmental, and social issues facing teens today. Second, to help parents and other family members understand more fully the role they play in the lives of their teenagers. Third, to provide definitive information on the importance of families' involvement in the education of their teens. These goals were defined against a backdrop of national research that clearly indicates that young adolescents are worried about a lack of guidance in education, in career planning, in forming adult values, and in assuming adult roles.

My goal for this book was to bring together all this information in a concise, accurate format. The topics reflect our changing society, and with it, the need for new information. We are busy people today, and we want our information in quick, easy bits. However, we also want it carefully researched, written, and easy to read. To create a text that meets these requirements, we drew on the expertise of over fifty reviewers—each with years of training and experience in his or her field. These reviewers took the chapters we sent, and modified, added to, and commented on the text. They urged us on if we left out even one idea that would help families raise healthy, successful teens. They commented if we wrote too much or too little, or without complete clarity. All of those who reviewed (and often helped us write the text) are listed in our "Acknowledgments" section. Contributors to each topic area are also acknowledged in the specific chapters on which they worked. I express my deepest thanks and appreciation to these talented, dedicated professionals who care so much about the health of young people today.

Our special thanks go to Don Sweeney and Pat Morgan at the Michigan Department of Community Health. Without their faith in us, this book would not have materialized.

The writer and editor of *Healthy Teens*, Jim McCarthy, deserves a special commendation for handling difficult subjects with grace and good taste. Marcia Rayner Applegate has my gratitude for taking responsibility for assisting in the writing and editing, formatting the book, and checking resources. Laura Linenfelser and Kathy Brennan of P.S. Abrams contributed their wonderful design ideas for the cover and title page, and for the format of the book.

With this printing in February, 1997, *Healthy Teens* is now published in its second edition. The first edition, published in August, 1996, sold out (15,400 copies) in just thirty days. We have used reactions from our readers to expand *Healthy Teens*. Several chapters have been expanded, and new sections on college financial aid, dyslexia, oral hygiene, and a full chapter on sexual harassment have been added. We sincerely thank several new reviewers for their help on these additions. We have also expanded our resource list, since we strongly believe this feature of the *Healthy Teens* is very important to families.

Alice R. McCarthy, Ph.D.

Chapter 1

TEENS AT HOME

Teen Development

If there is a one-word synonym for adolescence, it is the word *change*. Teens go through physical changes, changes in behaviors and beliefs, and changes in how they see themselves in the world at large and within their families.

Adolescent development has both its bright sides and its shadows. On the darker side, most teens experience adolescence as the most unhappy stage of their lives. They are going through tremendous changes, and moving toward different kinds of relationships. Before adolescence, friendships are mainly boy-boy, and girl-girl. As they enter the teen years, there is a new "opposite sex" orientation to teen relationships, and kids are not sure how to act. There are uncertainties of how to relate to others of the opposite sex, and how to handle friendships with those of the same sex. Many teens feel overwhelmed by new romantic and sexual feelings and impulses.

One reason that adolescence is such a time of stress between parent and child is that, in their unhappiness, teens lash out at the closest (and safest) victims—their parents. Another reason for parent-teen stress is that teens, in trying to relate to peers and not knowing how, may go overboard. Teens tend to think things like, "If I throw a big party, the other kids will accept me," or, "If my parents set rules for where I can go and how late I can stay out, the other kids will laugh at me."

On the brighter side, if your relationship with your child has been loving and appropriate during the pre-teen years, your child will have absorbed your values and ideals, and these won't change radically during adolescence. Then it is less likely that your child will get involved with kids who are bad influences—he or she will be attracted to friends who have values and ideals similar to the ones learned from you.

If you want to help your teen through adolescence, pay attention. Make sure you know where he or she is and what he or she is doing. It is not old fashioned to set a curfew. If your teen goes to a party, make sure the party is properly supervised by a responsible adult. Believe it or not, most teens like to feel that someone cares and is helping guide them through the strange landscape of the pre-adult wilderness. The teen years will end quickly enough, and most kids pass through them unharmed. As a parent, you can take courage in this, and remember that there is a lot you can do along the way to help.

Open Communication Channels

As a parent, you have daily opportunities to influence your teen's choices about life and health. The more you take those opportunities—if communication is a daily, ongoing process—the more influence you will have. If you talk to your teen about non-threatening subjects, if you watch television and movies together and share your ideas and values, you will be better able to talk over your concerns on serious subjects. If you have established a rapport, you and your teen will be more at ease, and will be able to talk without feeling uncomfortable. Your teen will be less likely to feel threatened, or feel that you distrust him or her.

If you do not have an open relationship with your teen, you may need to take some time to establish one. To start, show appreciation for positive behaviors and be a good listener when your son or daughter *does* talk to you. Ask questions to find out what your teen is truly interested in (even if you do not share the same enthusiasm), and encourage him or her to tell you about it.

How Families Can Help

You've shaken your head, had the arguments, questioned yourself, and have been through the trials and wonders of having a teenager in your home. What is important now is to know how to help your teen through the high school years and the more challenging aspects of adolescence. The following suggestions make a good foundation for a relationship between any two people, but are an especially important starting place for parents of a teen.

- Listen to your teen, even when you disagree. Try not to force your opinions on him or her.
- When addressing a problem, focus on specific behaviors that bother you instead of attacking basic personality traits or your teen's value as a human being. Don't confuse hating something your teen does with the love you have for your teen as a person.

- Don't nag or preach, and avoid constant criticism.
- Try to show your appreciation and love as often as possible.

You can be invaluable in helping your teen develop a realistic picture of himself or herself. In many instances, this is as simple as pointing out some of the obvious strengths of your teen—strengths that you both may take for granted or that may be clouded over by other events in your teen's life. This may be as easy as encouraging your teen in hobbies and helping him or her get involved in extracurricular activities at school. Try to help your teen see opportunities that he or she might enjoy and that might provide a chance for your teen to learn about himself or herself.

Another area that you can help your teen with is finding out about real-life job opportunities and careers. Beyond a job title, many teens don't really know what the adults in their lives do for a living. Here again, you can expand your teen's world, taking him or her beyond the relatively small world of family, school, and friends, to finding out more about the adult world, and discovering how he or she will fit in.

The Big Picture

In the largest sense, adolescence is about finding an identity, which requires a certain amount of trial and error at any age. Your role as a parent or caring adult is to help shepherd and support the adolescent experiment without turning your teen's adolescence into *your* experience, a part of *your* insecurities, or *your* unfinished business. Remember, you are the adult and your teen is still your child. For example, adults who over-identify with their child's search for identity—who react and overreact to every twist in the road and every challenge to what they think is best—can easily change a teen's search for identity into something that has more to do with the adult than the teen.

Some families are over-controlling of their teen. Letting go is never easy, but adolescence is a time for adults to give a teen space to grow. It is tempting to step in, trying to dictate solutions or find cures for personal problems. You may be offering a safety net that is, in reality, a smothering blanket.

Teens react to over-involvement and over-control in two fairly predictable ways. One way is to base their search for identity on being *against* everything their parents stand for. At just the opposite extreme are teens who decide to end—or never begin—their search for identity by letting the adults in their lives decide everything. In either case, the experience that is so important to discovery is lost. Teens lose, families lose.

Moving Beyond Adolescence

Think back to your own adolescence and your own high school years. Adolescence is a period most people think fondly about on occasion, but would never actually want to go back to. Your teen will probably feel the same way. The passions, the discovery of one's sexuality, the ups and downs, the special moments with friends, the triumphs and heartbreaks—at some point, give way to

a calmer breeze. One day—probably just as you did—your teen will return to you. He or she might not be the same person who "left," but the chances are that you will like and love him or her just as much or more.

Building Assets for Life

Search Institute, in Minneapolis, Minnesota, has identified "40 Developmental Assets for Youth" (see "Appendix A") that contribute to healthy development and eventual success in life. The more assets a child or teen has out of the forty, the more likely he or she will be able to succeed in society and in life.

The main idea behind Search Institute's asset-building program is that *everyone* in a community can be involved in fostering these assets in *all* children and teens, but if anyone plays lead in the asset-building band, it is the family. Without a strong family, it is much more difficult to nurture a solid foundation for development in children and adolescents. Parents and other caregivers who have begun using the asset-building approach find that it gives a concrete, sensible perspective for thinking about parenting and family life—beginning at birth and continuing through adolescence

Rather than offering a laundry list of "stuff you should do," the asset-building approach suggests priorities and perspectives to shape the parenting task. This framework offers several key benefits.

- *A focus for parenting*—The asset-building framework reminds parents of the "bottom line" in their child-rearing. Rather than focusing on

"getting ahead" or "avoiding problems," the assets help parents see that
their primary role lies in raising
caring, competent, and responsible
young people.

- *Affirmation and motivation*—Asset
building reminds parents that what
they do makes a big difference. Asset
building motivates parents to stay actively involved in their children's
lives through adolescence, rather than
assuming that teenagers no longer
need their parents when they are
becoming independent.
- *A positive perspective*—Many parent
educators say they struggle to get
parents to come to workshops because
parents are afraid of being labeled as
having problems with their kids. By
emphasizing the positive things all
young people need, asset building can
break down the barriers and reduce
the stigma of seeking support and
guidance.
- *Partners in parenting*—Because asset
building seeks to nurture a shared
responsibility in the community for
raising the youngest generation, this
approach promises to provide families
with a supportive, caring network of
partners in raising their children. In
short, it begins to recreate the kind of
informal community that previous
generations of parents depended on.

Asset building doesn't offer a neat set of
techniques and tricks for more effective
parenting. Rather, it provides parents
with some basic principles for making
decisions and shaping family life. There
will still be ups and downs. There will
still be challenges—and pain—but asset
building can help parents be intentional
about their choices, knowing that what

they do can have a tremendously positive
impact in shaping their children's lives.

A Guide to Teen Parties

Face it—parties have been a fact of life
for teens and families forever. The right
kinds of parties can be an important
factor in your teen's growth into adulthood. The planning of a party, and even
talking about going to parties, can help
build trust between you and your teen.
You also need to be aware of your
responsibilities—to your teen and to your
family—when your son or daughter wants
to go to a party or have a party at home.

When the Party Is at Your House

By high school, teens should be capable
of planning a party of their own. Your
responsibility is to set the broad guidelines for the party.

- No open houses and no crashing. You
need to make sure that your teen
understands that unwanted guests are
just that—*unwanted.*
- No smoking, alcohol, or drugs.
- House rules apply. Party or no party,
your teen needs to know that the standards of conduct you have set for
your household apply during a party.
- No wandering around the house or
leaving the party and coming back.
Teens should not have access to bed-
rooms or be allowed to wander
around your neighborhood.

You also need to know your own increasing responsibility for parties given
in your home. The two largest problems
are uninvited guests and the use of
alcohol and drugs, especially when there

is no adult at home during the party. Don't put the burden on your teen to be an adult and enforce the ground rules of the party. Your presence needs to be felt but not overbearing. Make sure that your teen knows that he or she can come to you for help if the party starts to get out of control.

It is against the law to allow anyone under 18 to smoke (in your home or otherwise), or to allow anyone under 21 to drink alcohol. Adults are legally responsible for anything that happens to a minor who has used alcohol or drugs in their home. Penalties can include jail time and fines (see "Appendix .C").

When Your Teen Goes to a Party

There are a few simple rules to follow if your teen wants to go to a party or dance or other social event.

• Know exactly where your teen is going and who he or she is going with.
• Know that adults will be present. If necessary, call and check.
• Know when the event starts and when it will be over.
• Know how your teen is getting to and from the event.

When you decide whether to let your teen socialize, consider two important factors: How willing is your teen to follow your guidelines? How willing are you to plan in advance with your teen to help him or her avoid or get out of bad situations?

Any rules you set should at least include an agreement to call home if anything

unusual comes up. This means that your teen knows that whatever happens—from needing a ride because a date has been drinking, to being drunk himself or herself—you will help out. For kids in high school, it is best to allow your teen to save face and agree to meet you a short distance away from the party or event. Make it easy for your teen to choose this option by agreeing not to punish or restrict your teen for whatever it is that happened.

When You're Away from Home

Unsupervised parties are never a good idea, whether at your home or someone else's. Your teen needs to know that you forbid parties while you are away because you will be held responsible for events that occur in your absence. Make sure your son or daughter understands that this is not a matter of trust between you. The facts are that it is a matter of your liability to other teens who may get in trouble at your house. Your teen also needs to know the dangers of attending parties where there is no adult supervision. Remind your teen of how quickly a bad situation can develop without any adults around. Finally, many of these problems become much less of an issue for adults who allow supervised parties in their home and allow their teen the freedom to go to supervised parties away from home.

Some high schools have family member meetings to help set up networking. If you have already had contact with the families of your son's or daughter's classmates, you may feel more comfortable contacting them when a party is planned. Teens also benefit because they know that adults are communicating with each other, and would be less likely to end up at "unauthorized" parties.

"Building Assets for Life" *adapted and reprinted with permission from* "Families Taking Action" *from* Healthy Communities: Healthy Youth *by Eugene C. Roehlkepartain and Peter L. Benson, Search Institute, Minneapolis, Minnesota.*

"Teen Development" *adapted from* You and Your Adolescent: A Parent's Guide for Ages 10-20, *by Laurence Steinberg, Ph.D., and Ann Levine.*

Contributions to and review of "Teen Development" *by:*

Eli Saltz, Ph.D., Director, The Merrill-Palmer Institute, Detroit, Michigan, and

Helene Mills, Ed.D., Principal, Seaholm High School, Birmingham, Michigan.

"Teen Development" reviewed by:

Stephen Spector, Ph.D., Psychologist, Beacon Hill Clinic, Birmingham, Michigan.

Donald B. Sweeney, M.A., Chief, School Health Unit, Community Public Health Agency, Michigan Department of Community Health, Lansing, Michigan.

Betty Tableman, M.P.A., Director, Prevention Services, Michigan Department of Community Health, Lansing, Michigan.

James Windell, M.A., L.L.P., Oakland Psychological Clinic, Oakland County Probate Court, Pontiac, Michigan.

Contributions to and review of "A Guide to Teen Parties" *by Helene Mills, Ed.D., Principal, Seaholm High School, Birmingham, Michigan.*

Chapter 2

TEENS, FAMILIES, AND SCHOOLS

Student Success

As the year 2000 and a new century approach, educators, schools, and community groups focus more and more on family involvement in education, and on school-family partnerships. Research supports two important conclusions. First, family involvement in a teen's school life means higher grades and higher test scores. Second, school-family partnerships mean higher graduation rates and higher rates of college attendance.

Below are three important facts for adults to consider.

- *Student achievement in school can be linked to practices at home*—A recent national study of 37 states showed that student absenteeism, the variety of reading materials available in the home, and excessive television watching accounted for nearly 90 percent of the difference in average state-by-state student performance.

- *What families do to help their children learn is more important to academic success than the family's financial status*—A national study showed that higher achievement in school across all academic areas is more the result of family involvement—especially in the area of completing homework assignments—than family financial status.

- *Families benefit from being involved in their teen's education*—The same study mentioned above found that family involvement in a teen's education, and school-family partnerships build self-esteem and help families develop stronger social ties to the community. Families learn more about schools, teaching and learning activities, and family members are more likely to pursue their own educational goals.

What Families Can Do

The basics of family involvement are simple. Make sure your child attends school regularly, encourage reading in the home, and limit television watching and video game playing. The suggestions below can help your teen's school performance even more.

- Encourage good study habits and help your teen keep track of—and complete—homework assignments.
- Stay informed about your teen's progress in school, especially through parent-teacher meetings.
- Set high standards for your teen. Encourage your son or daughter to take challenging classes and preparatory classes that may be prerequisites for higher level classes later on.
- Encourage your teen to participate in school extracurricular activities.

To be more effective and become actively involved, learn about your teen's school and school policies, get to know your teen's teachers and guidance counselor, support parent-teacher organizations, and serve on school volunteer boards that determine school policy, academic assessment, and/or curriculum development. Helping your teen *and* your family get the most out your teen's high school years requires a commitment by the family to the community at large.

School-Family-Community Partnerships

> The way schools care about children is reflected in the way schools care about the children's families. . . . If educators view students as *children*, they are likely to see both the family and community as partners with the school in children's education and development.
>
> *Joyce L. Epstein, Co-Director*
> *Schools, Family and Community*
> *Partnership Program*
> *Johns Hopkins University.*
> *Phi Delta Kappan, May 1995.*

Just about all families care about their children, want them to succeed, and are eager to obtain better information from schools and communities in order to remain good partners in their children's education. In surveys and studies involving teachers, parents, and students, some important patterns related to partnerships have emerged. Common themes are evident in successful programs. However, individual schools must tailor what they do to meet the needs and interests, time and talent, and ages and academic levels of students and families.

The "Six Types of Involvement" outlined in Tables 1, 2, and 3 in "Appendix B" include many different ways a partnership among students, parents, and schools can be set up. The tables provide examples of ways involvement can occur,

and the challenges ahead for schools, families, and communities.

Dr. Joyce Epstein of Johns Hopkins University has studied the hard work of many educators and families in many schools. She has learned that—along with clear policies and strong support from state and district leaders and school principals—an Action Team for School, Family, and Community Partnerships in each school is useful. She indicates that the action team guides the development of a comprehensive program of partnership, including all six types of involvement. The action team integrates the family and community connections within a single, unified plan and program.

The tables in "Appendix A" give just a hint of the exciting work ahead for schools, families, and communities that come together in a partnership to assist children's learning and development.

Dr. Epstein has established the National Network of Partnership 2000 Schools to help state, district, and school leaders who are ready to implement school/family/community partnerships. For an invitation and membership forms to join the Network, contact Dr. Epstein at The Center on Families, Communities, Schools and Children's Learning, Johns Hopkins University, 3505 N. Charles St., Baltimore, MD 21218, or call 410-516-8800.

Parent-Teacher Conferences

Many parents—and too many teachers—approach parent-teacher conferences with the kind of fear and dread usually reserved for root canals and IRS audits. Hopefully, the facts below will give you a fresh view and new optimism about parent-teacher conferences.

- *Most* teachers view parent-teacher conferences as a real chance to improve your teen's overall education and academic performance.
- Parent-teacher conferences are the single most important starting point for a working relationship between you, your teen's teacher, and your teen's school.
- Parent-teacher conferences are important at the high school level! More and more high schools are asking parents and other caring adults to attend conferences, and are scheduling conferences at more convenient times.

Getting Ready for Conferences

Talk with your teen before the conference. Put your teen at ease about the meeting by stressing that the conference is designed to make things better, not worse. You will want to discuss course work and homework, and ask if there is anything he or she would like you to discuss with the teacher.

Preparing for a parent-teacher conference serves two important functions. First, your questions, concerns, and hopes for your teen are all important to your teen's teacher. Second, being prepared can help put you at ease and help you and your teen's teacher set an effective agenda for the conference. Plan to be on time for the conference, and plan to end the conference on time. Plan to leave the conference with some specific next steps.

Before you go to the conference, jot down a few notes to yourself.

- Note anything about your family life, your teen, or your teen's habits or outside interests that you think might be important for the teacher to know.
- Note any questions you might have about your teen's progress.
- Note any questions you might have about the school's programs or policies.
- Write down ideas about how you, your teen, and the teacher can work together to enhance your son or daughter's education.

Once You're There

The questions below are adapted from an article written by Steven W. Enoch, a school system superintendent in California. The tips were originally written for teachers, but are presented here as questions for adults to ask of teachers. While this is not intended as a checklist, each question addresses a key point in your teen's educational development. Use them as a framework for your conference to provide a starting point for establishing an ongoing understanding with your teen's teacher.

- How are my teen's language skills developing in the areas of reading, writing, listening, and speaking? What can I do at home to help?
- In what areas is my teen making good academic progress? What areas need work?
- Can I see examples of my teen's work? (This can help illustrate and back up the teacher's feedback and evaluation.)

- Does my teen work well in group situations? Does my teen cooperate and interact well with others?
- Is my teen learning to think critically and creatively? In what ways?
- Can you give two or three specific goals to focus on that will help my teen develop academically?
- What kind of home practices will help my teens' academic work?
- Is there anything you need to know about my teen or my family in order to understand him or her better?

After the Conference

It is natural to judge your conference—on a scale of 1 to 10 or in simple words, like *good, indifferent,* or *bad*—and to want to reach some conclusions about your teen's school work as a result of the conference. You may even leave the conference angry or upset—feeling judged as a parent or caregiver—or feeling that the teacher did not see your teen in the right light. It is important not to spend too much time judging the conference or thinking your feelings toward your teen's teacher. Instead, plan how to use the conference to help improve your teen's academic life.

Here are some tips to help you use a single conference—regardless of how you feel about its outcome—to help your teen and build a continuing relationship with your teen's teacher and school.

- What did I learn that I need to discuss with my teen?
- What home practices do I need to start or improve that will help my teen?

- Do I need to schedule a follow-up conference with the teacher to discuss any unresolved issues?
- Do I need to schedule an appointment with my teen's guidance counselor in order to act on any of the information I learned?

Learning Differences

What is ADHD?

Attention-Deficit/Hyperactivity Disorder (ADHD) is a developmental disorder marked by three distinct behaviors.

- *Inattention*—Not knowing what task to attend to or not being able to stay focused long enough to finish a task.
- *Impulsivity*—Not being able to control urges to speak or act, and not thinking about the consequences.
- *Hyperactivity*—Excess physical movement, often without purpose or with a "driven" quality.

While some two million school-age children have ADHD, this disorder frequently persists into adolescence and adulthood. Treatment for ADHD is based on individual needs, and may include special schooling, individual and/or family counseling, and medication. Support groups are also available. Persons who exhibit the behavior patterns of ADHD should be evaluated by a professional skilled in working with the disorder. ADHD medications should be managed by physicians—typically psychiatrists and neurologists specializing in behavioral symptoms. Treatment for ADHD rarely includes medication alone.

What used to be called *ADD with hyperactivity* is now called ADHD. What used to be called *ADD without hyperactivity* is now called *ADHD, Predominately Inattentive Type*. Adolescents with the latter disorder are often described as lazy, "spacey," and unmotivated. As a general rule, girls suffer more commonly from the inattentive type, and effective treatment and support are difficult to obtain.

How ADHD Affects Teens

Simply put, adolescents with ADHD don't *do* the things they mean to do—or say they will do—and they *do* things or say things that they don't mean to. Such a simple description may seem unfair to teens and adults already faced with the disorder, or may seem so general as to fit almost every adolescent. For some families, this simple description is a beginning toward looking at difficulties that have been affecting a child and the whole family since the child was as young as three or four.

For adolescents with ADHD—diagnosed or undiagnosed—the disorder can spiral into chronic behavior problems at school and at home, and almost daily troubles with peers and authority figures. Adults often blame themselves for the disorder or think of their child as simply "bad." Besides the impact on families, the social cost ripples outward into society in the form of lost productivity, underemployment, re-education costs, drug and alcohol abuse, and even crime.

The American Psychiatric Association's *Diagnostical and Statistical Manual of Mental Disorders (DSM-IV)* includes standards for evaluating children for ADHD before the age of seven. Unfortunately, no single, authoritative criteria exists for evaluating adolescents who may have ADHD. The normal pressures of adolescence can also complicate the process of getting help for ADHD. Worse still, many families of children diagnosed with ADHD have adjusted—and/or maladjusted—to the disorder to such an extent that help may seem unreachable, if not downright out of the question. As you read, try to find the distance necessary from your everyday life to really think about your child and his or her behavior.

Above all, adults should resist putting questions like, "How was school today?" or "What grade did you get on the math exam?" before talking about how their teen *is* today. The following guidelines, developed by Lou Stewart, may help.

- Use a planner. Check off completed assignments and put them in a regular place to turn in the next day.
- Plan ahead. Organize homework and long-term assignments such as tests and term papers well beforehand.
- Check daily assignments with your teen. Emphasize planning when it comes to long-term assignments.
- Reward completed work and school success.

What is Dyslexia?

According to the U.S. Department of Health and Human Services, it is estimated that as many as 15 percent of American students have dyslexia.

Research experts believe dyslexia is a change in the brain structure that causes individuals to have difficulty with acquisition of language. As used here, "dyslexia" refers to a condition that causes individuals who exhibit average or above-average intelligence to have difficulty learning to read, write, spell, and comprehend as expected.

Dyslexia is not a disease. It is not "caught," nor is there a vaccination that will prevent it. Its causes are unclear, but dyslexia is not specific to age, gender, race, or ethnic background. The bad news is there is no cure for dyslexia. The good news is that dyslexia is a physiological or physical problem with an educational solution.

To most people, dyslexia simply means reading or writing backwards. People with dyslexia display a wide range of symptoms related to perception and learning. It is hard to believe that in this day of instant communication, little information has reached the average parent, teacher, physician, psychologist, or others in positions to help. This is true in spite of the fact that thousands of articles on dyslexia have been written, and successful teaching strategies to have been in use for sixty years. According to the National Institutes for Health, only ten percent of the teachers in our country are trained to teach students with dyslexia.

Dyslexia and School

Many teens with mild dyslexia are never identified, and therefore struggle through school. They may be described as "lazy," "not too bright," or "slow." The more severely affected students will be part of the bottom reading group and are often formally labeled "learning disabled." They frequently have feelings of being stupid or even retarded. Dyslexia may be a condition that was overlooked in your teen's earlier school years. The following list of symptoms may help you determine if your son or daughter is dyslexic.

- Average to above average intelligence.
- Difficulty in sounding out unfamiliar words.
- Difficulty with memory and recall of words in written and oral expression.
- Comparatively high frequency of reading, writing, and spelling errors, such as omissions, additions, substitutions, or reversals.
- Problems organizing, sequencing, and/or retrieving information.
- Difficulty following or remembering oral instructions.
- Reading, spelling, and/or comprehension skills which fall below expectation.
- Excelling in art, music, drama, mechanics, athletics, problem solving, or hands-on activities.

Related characteristics may include the following.

- Delayed speech development or speech problems.
- Left-handedness, or ability to use both hands (ambidexterity).
- Family history of language learning problems.
- Difficulty with math.
- Allergies.

- Attention Deficit Disorder with or without hyperactivity.
- Difficulty with abstract concepts of time and direction (left-right confusion).

People with dyslexia learn best when information is structured in a sequential fashion that moves from the simple to the complex. Knowledge about language and its rules need to be directly taught. For some, one-on-one instruction is essential. Seeing, saying, and doing (multi-sensory learning) is crucial. The first step in an instructional program is an approach called "synthetic phonics." The Orton-Gillingham teaching approach has been successful for thousands of people with dyslexia around the world.

Beyond Dyslexia

If a person with dyslexia fails often enough and is misunderstood, secondary emotional problems can arise which can further contribute to reading difficulties. Many grow up with self-doubts about their intelligence and ability. Frustration and disappointment in their educational, occupational, and personal achievements are common.

With family support and proper teaching, students with dyslexia can succeed in all walks of life. Many dyslexics excel in architecture, engineering, the arts, business, politics, and sometimes math and science. They often like and are good at hands-on activities. Some have the knack of seeing the "whole forest" while others are still "counting the trees." Famous people with dyslexic characteristics include Thomas Edison, Hans Christian Andersen, Albert Ein-

stein, General George Patton, Woodrow Wilson, Nelson Rockefeller, Bruce Jenner, Greg Louganis, Cher, Danny Glover, Henry Winkler, and Whoopi Goldberg.

If your teenager has many characteristics from the checklists, you should look into testing for dyslexia by a trained specialist in that field. It could be a psychologist, a school psychologist, a physician, or a language evaluator for dyslexia. If your school has no specially trained teachers available, look into outside help. There are organizations that can put you in touch with help in your area. Communicate the results of the testing to your teen's teachers to make them aware of your teen's strengths and weaknesses. By law, if a person is diagnosed with dyslexia, they have the right to certain accommodations and instruction. Inquire about untimed tests, oral examinations, and even bringing a tape recorder into the classroom. Teens with dyslexia can also take the ACT and SAT tests orally.

Most importantly, concentrate on your teen's strengths, and not his or her weaknesses. Your teen needs to understand that his or her brain is simply wired differently for language. Dyslexia is a learning *difference*, not a learning disability.

"School-Family-Community Partnerships" modified with permission from writings by Joyce L. Epstein, Co-Director, Schools, Family and Community Partnership Program, Johns Hopkins University, Baltimore, Maryland.

"Parent-Teacher Conferences" adapted and abbreviated with permission from "Taking Charge of Parent-Teacher Conferences" by Steven W. Enoch (Education Week, March 22, 1995). Reviewed by Steven W. Enoch.

Contributions to and review of "What is ADHD" *by Lou Stewart, M.A.T., L.D., diagnostician and educational therapist, Birmingham, Michigan.*

"What is ADHD?" *reviewed by:*

Stephen Spector, Ph.D., Psychologist, Beacon Hill Clinic, Birmingham, Michigan.

Betty Tableman, M.P.A., Director, Prevention Services, Michigan Department of Community Health, Lansing, Michigan.

Joel L. Young, M.D., Medical Director, Psychiatric Evaluation and Referral Center, Crittenton Hospital, Rochester, Michigan.

"What is Dyslexia?" *written by Laura Coens, Director of Communications, Michigan Dyslexia Institute/ Dyslexia Association of America.*

"What is Dyslexia?" *reviewed by*

John Howell, Ph.D., F/A.O.G.P.E., Director of Abrams Teaching Laboratory and Research, Michigan Dyslexia Institute/Dyslexia Association of America.

Kay Howell, M.A., F/A.O.G.P.E., Michigan Dyslexia Institute/Dyslexia Association of America.

Chapter 3

TEENS AND LIFE AFTER HIGH SCHOOL

The World of Work

When it comes to the world of work, teens usually hear what their elders heard—"Education is important—so study hard." Actually, it is not quite that simple. For example, who would have predicted the changes seen in recent years? New developments in technology—electronic devices unknown a decade ago—have had dramatic effects on everyday life. Massive corporate buyouts, drastic downsizings, and complete reorganizations have become commonplace. A growing number of people are deciding to leave the traditional corporate setting to work for or start smaller companies. Many opt to work on their own, in their homes, using computers to get the job done.

It is essential that teens get a realistic look at the world that is unfolding so that they can move forward, full of optimism and anticipation—prepared for and excited to join in the world of work. Here are significant factors to consider.

- The nature of global competition—the knowledge, skills, abilities, and attitudes necessary for success.
- The career or job search.
- The teen's role in self-development.
- The family's role in preparing teens for the future.

Jobs: Past and Future

Many of the jobs our parents performed are now obsolete or will be obsolete within the next decade. Jobs such as grocery store cashier, now being done by employees with scanners, will one day be done by the customer, much as we now have self-service gas pumps with credit card machines attached. As jobs become more and more automated, both the number of people needed and the skill levels of those employees are reduced. With the reduction in skills required comes a reduction in the salaries paid.

At the other extreme are jobs in computer technologies—from software programming and systems design and construction, to sophisticated medical equipment specialties. The complexity in many computer fields is so great and the skill levels so high, that those who can do the job are both in great demand and highly paid.

In his book, *The Work of Nations*, Robert Reich organized the jobs of the future into three categories.

- *Routine Production Services*—These jobs can be done by lower level employees anywhere in the world. Such jobs are in decline as automation and robots are replacing the need for human hands. This category includes word processing and the routine processing of medical claims at an insurance company. For example, English language textbooks are produced daily by non-English speaking workers in China.

- *In-Person Services*—Jobs included in this category are physical therapists and health care workers, beauticians, taxi cab drivers, and hotel workers. The job skills and pay vary by the complexity of the job.

- *Symbolic/Analytical Services*—These are the fastest growing jobs, the most challenging, and the highest paying. They include scientists, engineers, physicians, lawyers, bankers, real estate developers, consultants of all kinds, computer specialists, organization development specialists, strategic planners, recruiters, sales and marketing professionals, film editors and producers, writers, journalists, and musicians. These people spend most of their time conceptualizing problems, designing solutions, and implementing the required actions. Most have degrees—many have advanced degrees.

All of the jobs listed above can be done anywhere in the world—and they are—so the competition is not just the student sitting next to your teen, but students all over the globe. It is important that teens understand this new world competition so they can prepare for their place in the global economy.

A 1996 Michigan State University study of job prospects for the nation's graduating college seniors showed that a healthy economy predicted for 1997 will mean a stronger job market and increased job security for college graduates. The more than 500 employers surveyed anticipate a 6.2 percent increase in job prospects, which will sustain an expanding job market for four more years, according to the 26th annual *Recruiting Trends* study. The study showed shortages of computer science majors, programmers, systems

analysts, actuaries, transportation and logistics management majors, and electrical engineers.

Patrick Scheetz, director of Michigan State University's Collegiate Employment Research Institute, reports that things look better than they have in a decade (December, 1996). "I'd tell high school and college students to hang in there with the math and science classes," Scheetz said.

The box below lists the academic majors predicted to offer the five best and worst estimated starting salaries for 1996-97 college graduates.

Top five starting salaries	
Academic	**Estimated**
Major	**starting salary**
Chemical Engineering	$ 42,758
Mechanical Engineering	$ 39,852
Electrical Engineering	$ 39,811
Industrial Engineering	$ 37,732
Computer Science	$ 36,964
Bottom five starting salaries	
Liberal Arts/Arts & Letters	$ 24,081
Natural Resources	$ 22,950
Human Ecology/	$ 22,916
Home Economics	
Telecommunications	$ 22,447
Journalism	$ 22,102

Planning: A Critical First Step

Many working adults came by their jobs by the luck of the draw, with little or no planning. In many cases, the jobs offer little or no pleasure, use none of the person's natural skills, and, too often, are a drain on the emotional well-being of the individual and the family. The key phrase in this scenario is "little or no planning." You will want to help your teen formulate a plan—at the very least a direction—for his or her future work life.

The problem of choosing a career (for anyone) often seems too big to handle, but planning and breaking the problem down into tasks may help. Ask your teen the questions listed below, and then listen—really listen—to the answers.

- Identify your teen's personal goals and ambitions: What do they value most? What do they hope to accomplish?
- Identify strengths and natural talents. Where do they excel? Physical agility, science, math, English, music or theater, computers, communication skills, people skills (listening and/or teaching), and mechanical ability are some areas to explore.
- Identify career leanings. What would they do even if they weren't being paid? What particular tasks do they dislike, what tasks do they enjoy, and what activities do they absolutely love?

Once you find where your teen's interests and abilities lie, help and encourage him or her to research the jobs available. For a detailed listing of jobs, including duties, skills required, and salary ranges, see the *Occupational Outlook Handbook*. This reference offers descriptions of jobs most people have never heard of, and may help your teen decide on a career or a field of endeavor.

After a job or field has been selected, encourage your teen to talk to people who are already in that job or field. Many people are flattered and happy to discuss their careers with others. Don't be reluctant to ask. Many will be pleased to have your teen spend time in their office or factory.

Where to Get Help

- Your high school's counseling department or career planning assistance programs. Ask about tests that help determine students' interests and areas of competence.
- College or university career centers (most have library references available).
- Your state's unemployment office.
- U.S. Armed Services recruiting offices: Some offer the Armed Services Vocational Aptitude Battery (ASVAB), without obligation to enlist. This test shows areas of aptitude and high interest areas.
- Local or school library.
- Bookstores.
- Web sites and books listed in the Resource section under "College."

The Role of the Student

Just as it is clear that the nature of work and competition is changing, it should be clear that the student's role in preparing for work must also change. Some of the necessary skills, such as strong oral and written communications and advanced mathematics, must be supplemented by computer proficiency, team building skills, listening, and strategic thinking skills. It is up to the student, with family support, to demonstrate personal initiative in seeking out the knowledge or training he or she needs for personal growth.

Your high school may offer a work-for-credit program (co-op), internships, or vocational training programs in your teen's area of interest. Some cities receive funds from the Joint Training Partnership Act for summer employment (ages fourteen to twenty-one). Many community education programs and college continuing education (non-credit and credit) courses help individuals learn, develop, and refine the skills needed in the world of work. Real work experience—hopefully in an area of interest—will provide invaluable training for your teen. Even a fast food restaurant job teaches teens responsibility and provides experiences in taking direction and working cooperatively. Try to help your teen find more meaningful work after that first job experience.

The Role of the Family

Few discussions about the future are of greater concern—or cause more sleepless nights—than a teen's choice about what to do after graduation from high school. The decision can set the tone for a teen's entire adult life.

As parents or guardians, you can advise, suggest, encourage, or even cajole, but when the decision is finally made, it must be your teen's choice. Your responsibility and obligation is to do all you can to help your teen make an informed decision, considering all the relevant factors surrounding that choice.

What Are Employers Looking for When They Hire?

In the next decade and beyond, employers are going to be looking for people with ten special qualities. Can you find your teen in this list?

1. *Problem Solvers*—people who look for every option to solve a problem and don't go around complaining or blaming others.
2. *Sifters and Sorters*—people who use their brains to make sense of the puzzles in the workplace, who know how to research and apply what they learn.
3. *Heads That Focus on the Bottom Line*—workers who are out for results.
4. *People Who Speak and Write Well*—workers who can get their point across clearly using the best choice of words, correct grammar, and spelling.
5. *Team Players Who Can Listen*—people who work well with others, and want to help everyone win.
6. *People Who Welcome New Technologies*—workers who can figure out ways to use new technologies to reach the company's goals.
7. *Idea People Who Are Creative*—people who try new ways of getting the job done.
8. *Leaders Who Have Insight into What the Future May Bring*—people with self-confidence and pride in themselves and their own judgment.
9. *"Surfers on the Third Wave"*—learners who understand how fast change occurs and can handle it well.
10. *Organizers and Developers*—people who can motivate and manage others and are good at directing and producing the best products and services.

"What are Employers Looking for When They Hire?" *adapted with permission from "Where Do I Fit In?" from* The Pryor Report Management Newsletter, *October, 1994 (P.O. Box 101, Clemson, SC 29633; 1-800-237-7967).*

The College Decision

This section on college was inspired by an extensive series developed by Rusty Hoover of *The Detroit News*. Beginning on July 14, 1996, "Countdown to College" has followed high school senior, Jason Bloom of Bloomfield Hills, Michigan, and other students through the complicated, competitive admissions process. This series is designed to help students and parents navigate the college admission maze. *The Detroit News* will continue to publish "Countdown to College" through the 1996-97 school year. All of the information is available at the *Detroit News* web site at, http://www.detnews.com/1997/newsx/college/index.htm. Ms. Hoover can be contacted at 313-222-2744.

Ms. Hoover's excellent research provides reliable financial aid information for families. For *Healthy Teens*, important additions came from William T. Munsell, Director of Financial Aid at Lake Superior State University in Sault Sainte, Marie, Michigan. Definitive guidelines for federal and Michigan grants, loans, and scholarships are presented in the "Financial Aid" section, beginning on page 20.

Making the Choice

During the junior year in high school or early in the senior year, you will want to work with your teen to choose six or eight colleges to review and to which he or she wants to apply. Think about the quality and range of the academic programs offered, and your teen's special talents and skills. Consider the size of the

---

Signposts

FRESHMEN
- Plan tentative college-prep course schedule for next four years.
- Visit a local college and walk around to get a feel for the atmosphere.

SOPHOMORES
- Start browsing through your school's or local library's college guidebooks, attend a college fair, or surf the Internet.
- Send away for information from colleges you are interested in.

October
- Take the PSAT for practice.

JUNIORS
October
- Take the PSAT.

Spring
- Take the ACT or SAT I and SAT II subject tests.
- Make a preliminary short list of fewer than a dozen schools and visit as many as possible.

Summer
- Using your grade point average and test scores as guideposts, draw up your list of colleges and mail out requests for applications.

SENIORS
Fall
- Retake the ACT or SATs if not satisfied with your scores.
- Fill out your applications. Ask your English teacher or college counselor to proofread your essays. Give teachers plenty of time to write letters of recommendation by asking them early in the school year.
- Mail out completed applications.
- Wait.

Signposts is part of an occasional series, "The Road to College," developed by Ariana Cha, Staff Writer for the Detroit Free Press. Reprinted with permission from The Detroit Free Press, Sunday, December 29, 1996. Ms. Cha may be contacted at 313-223-4541 or cha@det-freepress.com.

college or university and its geographic location. The characteristics of the school, such as racial or religious diversity, campus politics, and fraternities or sororities may also be important.

Your teen's high school guidance counselor, guidebooks, and Web sites will be a big help (see extensive list under "College" in the Resources section of this book). Remember, you are busy, and your teen is *very* busy, but watch for filing dates and help keep the process on track. And this is important: Do not eliminate colleges on the basis of cost at this time, because your family may be able to receive financial aid awards.

Martin C. Jischke, president of Iowa State University, writing in *Best Colleges Guide*, published by U.S. News and World Report, had this to say to his son, a musician, as he considered colleges and universities.

> There are many fine colleges and universities in the United States. While we want you to choose the one that appears to meet your educational needs, recognize that there are likely quite a number of institutions that can provide a rich educational experience. The richness of your particular experience will depend in no small part on the commitment and enthusiasm you bring to your time in college—both in your classes and in extracurricular activities on and off campus.

Financial Aid

When your son or daughter begins applying to colleges, make sure he or she also completes the *Free Application for*

> ### Need-Blind and Full-Need
> Colleges and universities are said to be "need-blind" if they accept students without looking at ability to pay as a criteria. Institutions are "full-need" if they will meet all demonstrated need. Many, such as Columbia University, are both need-blind and full-need. Be sure to ask before applying. Most of Michigan's fifteen public colleges and universities are need-blind, but not full-need.

Federal Student Aid (FAFSA) and other financial aid forms required by the college. These forms must be completed well in advance of the financial aid deadlines. Missing a deadline by only one day can cost your family thousands of dollars in scholarships and other forms of financial aid. For example, the 1997-98 deadline in Michigan for the FAFSA is February 21, 1997. Students who qualify for the Michigan Competitive Scholarship should always submit the FAFSA prior to the earliest deadline of the schools they are considering.

It is wise to file the FAFSA even though you have not completed your final income tax return. Estimated income figures may be used and corrected later. Families who wait beyond April 15 will likely have missed many financial aid opportunities.

Some families choose not to file the form each year their student is in college. This is a mistake. Income is only one of the factors used to determine a student's financial aid eligibility. For example, the number of family members attending college, business losses, and high family medical expenses are all taken into account in determining eligibility.

Contact the counseling department of your school or college for more information on qualifying for financial aid.

In addition to applying for federal, state, and college-sponsored scholarships and grants, check with the service clubs in your community for the possibility of obtaining a scholarship application. Three national groups that offer scholarships are the American Association of University Women (AAUW), the American Business Women's Association (ABWA), and Soroptimists International. You may want to check with your local Lions Club, Kiwanis Club, or Rotary Club, as well. Criteria for these awards can vary.

Private scholarships are available from a variety of sources (listed in several books and on Web sites). Beware of scholarship services that guarantee a scholarship for a hefty fee. Scholarship scams have become much more prevalent recently, and the Federal Trade Commission (FTC) has become very aggressive in prosecuting offenders. The National Fraud Information Center may be contacted at 1-800-876-7060.

Federal Financial Aid

Federal financial aid programs provide nearly 70 percent of financial aid funds, colleges and universities provide 20 percent, and state and private sources provide 10 percent. Seek out information on financial aid sources early in the financial aid process to obtain a basic understanding of the programs and eligibility criteria.

Almost all federal aid is driven by the FAFSA. This form will tell you whether your teen qualifies for a subsidized or unsubsidized loan. As a general rule of thumb, students don't have to pay back grants or scholarships. Students do have to pay back loans. Several federal programs are described below.

- *Stafford Loans*: These are federal loans that come in subsidized and unsubsidized versions. The government picks up the interest on subsidized Stafford loans while the student is enrolled at least half-time in school. On unsubsidized loans, the interest accumulates while the student is in school, though the payments can be deferred until the student is out of school. While subsidized loans go to needy students, those who have no need can get an unsubsidized Stafford loan. Interest rates are capped at 8.25 percent.
- *Perkins Loans*: Designed for high-need students, these subsidized loans make up the best loan package available for students. Interest is capped at 5 percent.
- *Pell Grants*: These outright gifts are designed for students with high need. There are no academic criteria for these grants. The student must demonstrate need and be enrolled in an eligible institution. The maximum grant for 1997-98 is $2,700.
- *Supplemental Educational Opportunity Grants (SEOG's)*: These grants don't have to be paid back, are targeted to high-need students, and they are not based on merit.
- *Federal Work-Study Program*: Colleges are awarded funds that the student can earn by working in such areas as food service, the library, computer center, or offices. These

programs are based on need. The student earns the amount of the aid by working while attending school, and this money does not have to be paid back after graduation.

- *Americorps*: A federal community service program in which volunteers receive living allowances and contributions for college costs for 1,700 hours of annual service. For information, call 1-800-942-2677.
- *PLUS Loan*: Most families are eligible for the federal PLUS Loan which provides financial assistance to make up the difference between the student's cost of education and the financial aid received. The interest rate is variable, with a cap of 9 percent and a minimum monthly repayment of $50. Detailed information on the PLUS Loan may be obtained by writing to or calling the Federal Student Aid Information Center (P.O. Box 84, Washington, DC 20044-0084; 1-800-433-3243).

Michigan Financial Aid Programs

- *Michigan Competitive Scholarship*: These scholarships are for students who are Michigan residents, attend a Michigan public or private college or university, and who achieve a qualifying score on the ACT. For 1996-97, qualifying students had scores of greater than 90 for the sum of the ACT subtests. Scholarships range from $100 to $1,000 at public colleges, or $2,300 at private schools (awards are based on demonstrated financial need).
- *Michigan Tuition Grants*: These grants are awarded to students with

financial need who are going to private Michigan colleges. Scholarships range from $100 to $2,300, based on demonstrated financial need.
- *MI-LOAN*: This is a loan program for students attending Michigan colleges and universities. This loan is attractive because it allows for the possibility of up to five years of interest-only payments in the fifteen-year repayment period (non-need-based). Applicants must pass credit checks—parents often co-sign.
- *TIP (Tuition Incentive Program)*: TIP pays tuition and mandatory fees for associate degrees or certificate program courses for students from low-income families at community colleges and some four-year universities, including Michigan State University and Michigan Technological University. If a student earns an associate degree through the TIP program, TIP may provide up to $2,000 for students pursuing a bachelor's degree at a Michigan school. Students who are receiving or have received Medicaid from the Michigan Family Independence Agency are eligible. Students must apply before graduating from high school or receiving a General Education Diploma (GED), and be under the age of twenty at the time of high school graduation or GED completion. (1-800-243-2847; 7:30 a.m. to 4:30 p.m., weekdays).

Please check the Resources section of *Healthy Teens*, under "College," for further help on financial aid (web sites and books are listed). For financial aid in Michigan, contact the *Michigan Higher Education Assistance and Student*

Loan Authorities (1-800-877-5659; 7:30 a.m. to 5:00 p.m., weekdays), or the *Michigan Higher Education Assistance Scholarships and Grants Office* (1-517-373-3394; 8:00 a.m. to 5:00 p.m., weekdays).

Information on scholarships can be obtained free on the Internet or in libraries, or at a nominal cost from the state's MI-CASHE Scholarship Search Service.

For specific information on college and university standards in Michigan, see "Appendix D."

"The World of Work" *section was developed by Joseph Malgeri, M.S.M., Career Solutions, Troy, Michigan. This section was modified for the second edition printing.*

Special thanks to Rusty Hoover, Staff Writer for the Detroit News.

Contributions to and review of college financial aid information by William T. Munsell, Director of Financial Aid, Lake Superior State University, Sault Sainte, Marie, Michigan.

Chapter 4

TEENS AND PHYSICAL HEALTH

Building an Active Lifestyle

The high school years are a crucial time in the development of a person's attitudes and habits about physical activity and fitness. Teens' bodies are maturing into adulthood, and lifelong habits are taking root. As with other aspects of a child's or teen's life, adult family members help set the direction for life choices concerning fitness. The family can continue to use influence in directing their teen toward a healthy lifestyle by giving the proper message, both by example and by encouragement. Teens need to learn that physical activity is important now, and throughout their lifetimes.

Many of the activities of modern life provide little or no physical movement, such as sitting at a desk or computer, driving in a car, playing video games, or watching TV. Therefore, caring adults need to emphasize that physical activity must be sought out consciously. Adults need to set a clear, healthy example.

Physical Activity and Health

Though the importance of physical activity to good health has long been known, evidence continues to mount. Some evidence is highly encouraging, such as new research that shows that physical activity can help ward off and alleviate depression, and that vigorous physical activity by teenage girls can build strong bones, and prevent bone loss later in life. Some evidence is frightening, such as statistics that show that preventable chronic diseases and injuries will shorten the lives of *nearly 50 percent* of Michigan children. Two major factors contributing to these chronic diseases are inactivity and excess weight. Altogether, poor diet and lack of physical activity will result in more deaths than alcohol, firearms, infections, poisons, irresponsible sexual behavior, motor vehicles, and illicit drug use combined.

The Bad News

- Physical inactivity is the *single largest* risk factor for chronic disease.
- Overall, two out of three high school students do not meet the minimum national standard for physical activity of at least three 20-minute sessions weekly.
- Recent studies have shown that one in three Michigan school children are significantly overweight.
- Four out of ten school children in Michigan have high cholesterol levels.
- High blood pressure starts early for many kids: It affects one out of twelve Caucasian youth and one out of six African-American youth.

High school students need to get the serious message about the health risks of an inactive lifestyle. Teens will benefit by seeing the adults in their lives taking physical activity seriously. If adults don't take positive actions for their own health and fitness, the children and teens who live with them may wonder just how important physical activity and fitness are, and draw their own conclusions that physical activity and good health are not important.

The Good News

- A regular routine of physical activity is a simple remedy for potentially serious health problems later in life.
- Exercise has been shown to benefit both physical and mental health.
- Regular physical activity is great family fun. Exercising with your kids at any age is a good thing to do, whether it is just taking a walk, sharing a game of one-on-one, or spending some weekends and vacations doing outdoor activities.
- For individuals who are overweight, consistent physical activity can improve health risk factors and self-esteem, even without weight loss.
- It is never too late to start good health and fitness habits.

Competitive Sports

Organized sports will always be popular, and may provide a high level of fitness and well-being for those who participate. Team sports let kids see that physical fitness and skill can be important as routes to self-esteem and popularity. But the competitive nature of sports may give the message that these benefits are not for everybody. There is a danger that the overall message kids get is that physical fitness is primarily about competition, and that only the best are allowed to participate. With this focus, even student athletes run the risk of losing the motivation to seek out physical activity once their competitive careers are over.

Those who do not participate, whether it is because they are less physically gifted

or just aren't as interested, may turn into spectators, ready for a lifetime of watching sports on TV and from the stands.

Lifetime Fitness

All kids, especially those who do not participate in competitive sports, need positive messages and examples about physical activity intended to promote *lifetime fitness*. School physical education classes, which traditionally provided exercise and training for public school students, are now serving fewer than one third of high school students. Even for those enrolled in physical education, classes may not be long or frequent enough to provide needed levels of physical activity. Therefore, family and personal motivation is vital.

Teens may choose to engage in individual or group activities such as walking, jogging, weight training, aerobics, hiking, bicycling, rollerblading, and swimming. They may enjoy movement disciplines such as dance, yoga, or tai chi, and martial arts such as aikido, judo, or karate. One caution for weight training: Unsupervised strength training can result in significant harm to the musculoskeletal system in growing children. Teens should be taught correct warm-up, cool-down, stretching, and breathing techniques.

Each individual needs to find physical activities that he or she enjoys. Families and schools need to encourage every child and adolescent to do just that. The issue of lifelong health is simply too serious to allow teens to slide by without a physical activity plan that includes a minimum of 30 minutes a day of activity which increases the heart rate and breathing, plus more vigorous activity at least three days a week.

The Michigan Governor's Council on Physical Fitness, Health, and Sports is making a concerted effort to promote fitness among citizens of Michigan. Their booklet, "Let's Take a Walk" and other information on health and fitness can be obtained free of charge by calling the Health Promotion Clearinghouse at 1-800-537-5666.

In its position paper, *The Importance of Physical Activity for Children and Youth*, The Governor's Council states:

> Perhaps the most important source of learning is from family members. Parents who do not engage in physical activity place their own health in jeopardy, but more importantly, miss an opportunity to be solid role models for their children. It is recommended that parents make family "policies" that include daily physical activity that is enjoyable for all family members.

Healthy Eating

Teens are notorious for eating half meals, eating on the run, consuming large quantities of fast food, snacking on fatty, sugary, or salty foods, and for skipping meals altogether. Try not to make food a power struggle. Eating is one of the few issues a teen can exert control over. Hopefully, the influence you have had on your teen's food habits and choices before the teen years will survive.

The core of the issue is to help your family develop healthy eating habits, not just for today, but for a lifetime. There *is* a link between what you eat and how you feel, how you look, and how you act now and in the latter years. Eating choices are extremely important. Diet-related diseases such as heart disease, certain types of cancer, and osteoporosis (brittle bones from lack of calcium) are related to food choices.

Teens generally do not see or care about "down the road" diseases. The challenge to the person in charge of food shopping and preparation is to be creative without the family knowing that they are eating for good health!

Food for families needs to come each day from the five food groups found on the Food Guide Pyramid. If families can possibly pay attention to the number of servings suggested for each food group, they will do fine. When you go to the grocery store, keep in mind that although prepackaged foods make life easier for busy families, they also contain more sodium (salt), refined carbohydrates, and fat than foods that you prepare yourself (besides generally costing more).

To help your family stay on a healthier diet, plan ahead so there are plenty of healthy snacks available.

- Fresh fruits and vegetables—cleaned, cut, and ready to eat.
- Low-fat dips.
- Low-fat crackers or pretzels.
- Low-fat popcorn.
- Low-fat chips and salsa.
- Low-sugar juices ready to drink.

Listed below are some more healthy snacks with the calorie count for each.

Food	Calories
1 cup blueberries	80
50 small, unsalted pretzels	50
1 rice cake	35
3 graham crackers (2½-inch sq.) .	90
2 cups cauliflower with 1 Tbl. reduced-calorie dressing	27
1 frozen fruit bar	70
1 nonfat blueberry yogurt (4.4 oz.)	50
1 cup minestrone soup	85
1 box minipack raisins (½ oz.) . . .	40
1 slice raisin bread with 2 tsp. light cream cheese	85
2 thick-style crispbreads	70
1 medium orange	60
1 small banana, wrapped in foil and frozen	99
1 fresh pear	98
10 cucumber slices topped with sliced mozzarella cheese (½ oz.) . . .	48

In addition to having poor eating and snacking habits, teens often skip breakfast. Research has shown that kids who do not eat breakfast do not do as well on tests in school. Their bodies have no "fuel" to go on! As an alternative, offer easy, "grab and go" foods to your teen.

- A sandwich.
- Cold pizza.
- Pudding.
- Pita bread or bagels.
- Frozen dinners that are low in fat and sodium.
- A milk shake.
- Leftovers of any kind.

Food Labels

Preparing a healthy diet is getting easier. manufacturers are required by law to label foods with their nutritional values. On each label, you will see a percentage of Daily Value listed for certain nutrients found in the food. The percent tells you how much of the maximum daily amount one serving contains. The percentages are based on the Daily Values for a 2,000-calorie diet. If a person needs fewer or more calories each day, decrease or increase the Daily Values slightly.

For Vitamins A and C, calcium, and iron, the Food and Drug Administration (FDA) considers any food that contains 10 to 19 percent of the Daily Value per serving a good source for that nutrient. If a food contains 20 percent or more of the Daily Value, it is an excellent source of the nutrient. Try to meet or exceed 100 percent of the Daily Value of these vitamins and minerals in the foods eaten each day.

With fat (especially saturated fat), sodium, and cholesterol, you want to look for lower percentages or levels. As a precaution, many foods labeled "no fat" or "low fat" may contain high levels of sugar and carbohydrates which may result in excess calorie intake.

When shopping for your family, remember that for the Daily Value of nutrients (per serving), 5 percent or less of saturated fat, 7 percent or less of cholesterol, and 6 percent or less of sodium are considered low, and better for good health.

Here is a sample nutrition label from a package of frozen vegetables.

Nutrition Facts

Serving Size ⅔ cup (89g)
Servings Per Container about 3

Amount Per Serving	
Calories 70	Calories from Fat 5

	% Daily Value*
Total Fat 0.5g	1%
Saturated Fat 2.5g	0%
Cholesterol 0mg	0%
Sodium 105mg	4%
Total Carbohydrate 12g	4%
Dietary Fiber 4g	16%
Sugars 6g	
Protein 5g	

Vitamin A 6%	•	Vitamin C 15%	
Calcium 0%	•	Iron 4%	

*Percent Daily Values are based on a 2,000 calorie diet. Your daily values may be higher or lower depending on your calorie needs:

	Calories	2,000	2,500
Total Fat	Less than	65g	80g
Sat Fat	Less than	20g	25g
Cholesterol	Less than	300mg	300mg
Sodium	Less than	2,400mg	2,400mg
Total Carbohydrate		300g	375g
Dietary Fiber		25g	30g

Calories per gram:
Fat 9   •   Carbohydrate 4   •   Protein 4

With food labels now listing nutrition facts, the choice is up to you whether to purchase a food or not.

Changing Needs for Growing Kids

Adolescents have increased nutrient needs because of the growth spurt that occurs during this stage of life. This growth spurt usually begins for girls around ages 10½ to 13½ years (with the highest rate being around ages 12 to 13), and for boys around the ages of 12½ to 15½ years (with the highest rate between ages 14 and 15).

Hormonal changes and the later onset of the growth spurt in boys contribute to greater muscle and skeletal growth, requiring a higher intake of protein, iron, calcium, and zinc. In contrast, the growth spurt in girls is characterized by a smaller increase in muscle mass and a greater increase in fatty tissue. The nutritional needs for girls are therefore somewhat lower than those for boys, except girls require more iron because of the onset of menstruation.

How adolescents feel about their bodies is closely related to how they feel about themselves. It is important for a teenager to know that change is normal. Reinforce for your teens that they need to take care of the body they have. Teens should be encouraged to talk about how they feel about their developing bodies with a supportive family member or a person they trust, such as a teacher or school counselor.

Vital Nutrients

Aside from seeing that your teen eats a relatively balanced diet from the five major food groups (see Food Guide Pyramid), the three most important nutritional requirements to monitor for teens are protein, calcium, and iron.

Protein—Many older teenage boys (ages 15 to 18) eat twice the recommended allowance of protein, or more, in the belief that a diet high in protein will give them a competitive advantage in sports. Misconceptions about the role of diet are common in the competitive world of sports. However, the basic facts are simple: Fitness and good performance require an adequate intake of calories and nutrients. With a few minor exceptions, eating enough from the five food groups on the Food Pyramid provides the proper intake; supplements and special preparations are generally unnecessary and may, in some instances, be harmful. Once the body's requirements for protein have been met, excess protein is processed just like any other excess form of calories—it is deposited as fat, not muscle. In addition, chronic excess protein consumption may have adverse effects on kidney function in the long term.

If your teen has decided to become a vegetarian, time will need to be spent making protein pairs (example: beans and rice) so he or she gets the amount of protein needed. Your library has numerous books available on healthy vegetarian eating. (Please see Resources.)

Calcium—As your teen's skeletal mass (size of bone structure) increases, his or her calcium requirements also increase. If calcium intake is very low, the body maintains normal blood-calcium levels by drawing calcium from the bones. This can have serious consequences: Teens may not develop optimal bone density, which may increase their susceptibility to the disease, osteoporosis, later in life.

Girls typically have too low an intake of calcium throughout the teen years, largely because milk—our single best source of calcium—is so often shunned as fattening. Skim milk is a good, low-fat source of calcium—a fact surprisingly few people realize. Teens who do not drink milk should be encouraged to include other the good sources of calcium listed here in their diet.

If you want a nutritious snack for non-milk drinkers, try this recipe.

Orange Julius Drink
1 can frozen orange juice (6 oz.)
1 cup milk
1 cup water
1 teaspoon vanilla
1 tablespoon sugar
10-12 ice cubes

Put all ingredients into a blender and blend until the mixture looks like a slush drink. This can also be frozen and eaten later as a popsicle-type snack.

Another reason for low calcium intake is the substitution of soft drinks for milk. If a fight develops over "no soft drinks in this house"—your teen will likely just get soft drinks from other sources. The trick is to think of ways to increase calcium, and it is strongly recommended that the calcium be provided in *food*, if at all possible. Check with your physician about a supplement if your teen does not drink any milk or eat any dairy products.

Other Sources of Calcium

Low-fat yogurt or cheese.

Add non-fat dry milk to meat loaf or hamburgers.

Calcium-fortified foods and drinks.

Calcium-precipitated tofu.

Canned salmon and sardines that contain the bones.

Iron—Iron requirements increase in adolescence because of the greater muscle mass and blood volume associated with the growth spurt. Refer to the Recommended Daily Allowances (RDA) chart on the next page for ages eleven to eighteen to help plan for the amount your teen needs. The onset of menstruation slightly increases the iron requirements for girls. Iron found in red meats (heme iron) is absorbed more easily than iron from grains and vegetables (non-heme iron). Consumption of vitamin C along with grains and vegetables will help with the absorption of non-heme iron, and will also increase the absorption of heme iron.

Teenagers may have difficulty obtaining the recommended 12-15 milligrams of iron a day from food sources alone if their calorie intake is low. Therefore, adolescents need to consume foods with a high availability of iron, such as red meats, or eat combinations of good non-heme sources of iron along with foods rich in vitamin C. An example would be, iron-fortified cereal with orange juice and/or an egg with orange juice. Your

physician can advise you about supplements to avoid iron deficiency anemia, if necessary.

Vitamins—The recommended vitamin allowances for adolescents can be comfortably met by a well-balanced diet.

Planning Family Meals

The Food Pyramid and the 1995 U.S. Dietary Guidelines that follow contain information that will help you in planning daily meals, and will guide your family, including your teen, toward a lifetime of healthy eating. Try to steadily adjust your family's diet toward a simple, balanced, no-nonsense routine of making healthier food choices.

1995 U.S. DIETARY GUIDELINES

- Eat a variety of foods.
- Balance the food you eat with physical activity—maintain or improve your weight.
- Choose a diet low in fat, saturated fat, and cholesterol.
- Choose a diet with plenty of grain products, vegetables, and fruits.
- Choose a diet moderate in sugars.
- Choose a diet moderate in salt and sodium.

RECOMMENDED DAILY ALLOWANCES AGE 11 TO 18

NUTRIENT		GIRLS		BOYS	
		11-14 years	15-18 years	11-14 years	15-18 years
PROTEIN	(g.)	46	44	45	59
CALCIUM	(mg.)	1200	1200	1200	1200
IRON	(mg.)	15	15	12	12

The Food Guide Pyramid

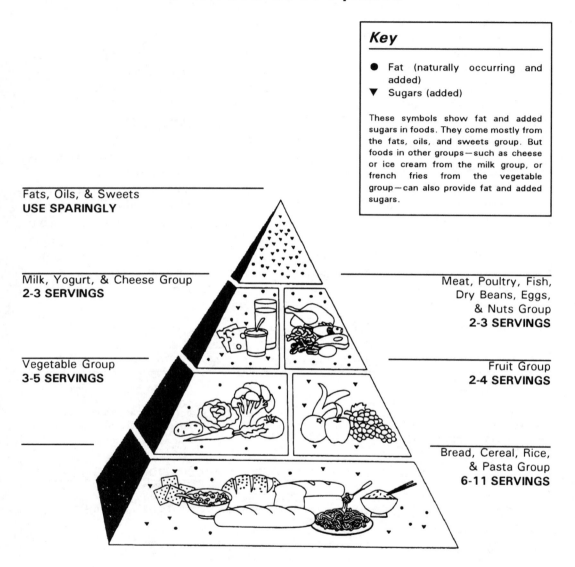

Key

● Fat (naturally occurring and added)
▼ Sugars (added)

These symbols show fat and added sugars in foods. They come mostly from the fats, oils, and sweets group. But foods in other groups—such as cheese or ice cream from the milk group, or french fries from the vegetable group—can also provide fat and added sugars.

Fats, Oils, & Sweets
USE SPARINGLY

Milk, Yogurt, & Cheese Group
2-3 SERVINGS

Meat, Poultry, Fish,
Dry Beans, Eggs,
& Nuts Group
2-3 SERVINGS

Vegetable Group
3-5 SERVINGS

Fruit Group
2-4 SERVINGS

Bread, Cereal, Rice,
& Pasta Group
6-11 SERVINGS

Looking at the Pieces of the Pyramid

The Food Guide Pyramid emphasizes foods from the five major food groups shown in the three lower sections of the Pyramid. Each of these food groups provides some, but not all, of the nutrients you need.

Foods in one group can't replace those in another. No one of these major food groups is more important than another—for good health, you need them all.

Eating Disorders

The "ideal" body—the body seen on television, in advertisements and fashion magazines, in athletics and in movies—can only be achieved by one percent of the population. This manufactured myth of the "perfect" body is often underweight and, in many cases, achieved through plastic surgery. Unfortunately, it is also sought by far more people than can ever achieve it. Recent studies show that one in ten college students—mostly young women—suffer from an eating disorder; either anorexia, bulimia, or binge eating. In some cases, the disorder had gone undetected since high school or even junior high.

It is impossible to place all the blame for eating disorders on the media or society at large. Personality traits such as a need for control or a perfectionist attitude, wider concerns of family life or relationships outside the family, or even hereditary factors may also play a role in eating disorders.

Anorexia nervosa can be simply defined as fat phobia—being afraid of becoming fat. Teens with this disorder often strive for perfection and control over their lives by controlling their body weight. Typically, these teens see themselves as fat well past the point when most others see them as thin to the point of being ill. Dangerous weight loss behaviors, continual dieting, and simply refusing to eat are the hallmarks of this disorder.

Bulimia is a binge and purge syndrome. Teens suffering from bulimia frequently eat very large amounts of food followed by getting rid of the food by excessive physical activity, vomiting, or using laxatives. For bulimics, food is a source of comfort and security, and a barrier against insecurity or depression.

Binge eating may well be the most common eating disorder. In this case, binges are not followed by purges, and the person typically becomes obese. Binge eaters may lose great amounts of weight by dieting, sometimes up to 100 pounds, but usually regain the weight quickly if there is no change in how they view themselves and how they eat.

Eating disorders are serious. If left untreated, eating disorders can lead to obesity, skin irritations and deterioration, hair loss, and much worse, irreversible health damage such as stunted growth, thinning bones, damage to teeth and internal organs, and the inability to reproduce. Studies show that between 10 and 15 percent of young people with anorexia nervosa or bulimia die from complications of the disease.

Adults also need to know that teens with eating disorders are usually very secretive about their eating habits. Shame and guilt keep teens (and adults) from talking about an eating problem to the people they love the most. The most obvious signs of an eating disorder already well in progress are listed below.

- Eating in private, or having strange eating habits.
- Eating much less than usual and skipping meals.
- Loss of energy or serious fatigue.

- Light-headedness, dizziness, or fainting.
- Lack of physical growth.
- Loss of menstruation.
- Extreme weight loss or weight gain.
- Difficulty swallowing or keeping food down.
- Excessive tooth decay or loss of tooth enamel.
- Damage to the throat from repeatedly vomiting.

The following questions are designed to help you recognize an eating disorder before the disorder has advanced. If possible, discuss these questions with your teen. You may even wish to modify the questions to ask younger children, especially pre-teens just entering junior high. *Yes* answers to the questions below—whether based on your observations or told to you by your teen—indicate a possible eating disorder.

- Does your teen eat far less than usual or skip two or more meals a day?
- Does your teen want to eat alone or in private?
- Does your teen have new, seemingly strange eating habits?
- Does your teen eat a large amount of food within a two-hour period, often seeming out of control in their eating?
- Does your teen eat large amounts of food when not hungry?
- Does your teen use laxatives, vomiting, excessive exercise, or other purging behavior to lose or control weight?
- Does your teen avoid social situations or stay at home to maintain an eating or exercise schedule?
- Does food seem to control your teen?

- Does your teen seem disgusted, depressed, or guilty after overeating?

Given the seriousness of eating disorders and the secrecy that usually goes with an eating disorder, adults frequently need to be the first to seek help for their teen. The help you seek needs to include medical and mental health professionals. However, a call to your school nurse or personal physician is usually a good starting point.

Dental Health

During the teen years, many young people begin neglecting the necessary care of their teeth. When children are younger, families often take responsibility for making sure they brush and floss regularly. As they become teenagers, older family members tend to assume that kids can handle this responsibility themselves, and no longer reinforce the need for good brushing and flossing.

Teens often develop extreme inflammation of the gums and an increased possibility of decay. Families often pay less attention to the diet of teens as well, so it is not unusual to see a big increase in tooth decay (cavities). Ask for advice from your dentist on how to keep track of your child's dental health, and for information on how you can help motivate your teen to take proper care of teeth and gums.

Preventing Injury

Many teenagers are active in sports and other physical activities and, as they get older, the amount of physical contact increases. Unfortunately, injuries can and do occur in sports, and they often involve the mouth—sometimes damaging teeth for a lifetime. While teeth can usually be restored to an acceptable function and appearance, the effects of dental injury are often lifelong. In order to prevent these devastating injuries, teen athletes should wear a mouthguard during sports or physical activities.

Mouthguards have traditionally been reserved for football or hockey, but today, mouthguards are also used for basketball, soccer, and field hockey. Both boys and girls now wear mouthguards during many sports activities. Ask your dentist to help you select a mouthguard that will best fit your son or daughter and adequately protect his or her teeth.

Orthodontics: A Lifetime Benefit

Orthodontics, usually called "braces," are recommended for many different reasons, and many teens need such treatment. When your dentist refers your child to the orthodontist, he or she is doing so for a specific reason. Most often, the reasons are related not so much to appearance but to the proper functioning of the teeth. Of course, after treatment they may also have nicer looking teeth due to a more correct positioning. When teeth are positioned correctly, the teeth and gums are healthier and easier to clean. These benefits will last for a lifetime.

If your son or daughter has braces, cleaning of the teeth and gums is extremely important. With wires, brackets, or appliances, it is more difficult to brush, and almost impossible to floss. Food also tends to collect on the brackets and bands, making more potential areas for decay to begin. The only solution is to take the extra time to make sure he or she maintains proper oral hygiene. This is difficult in the teenage years—a time when even toothbrushing is sometimes neglected. Both your dentist and orthodontist can help work with your teen on good home care, but they will need your participation to reinforce the importance of good dental hygiene habits.

Contributions to and review of "Building an Active Lifestyle" by Karen Petersmarck, M.P.H., Ph.D., Consultant, Division of Injury, Violence, and Surveillance, Michigan Department of Community Health, Lansing, Michigan.

Contributions to and review of "Healthy Eating" by:

Lois Thieleke, M.S., Extension Home Economist for Michigan State University Extension, Oakland County, Michigan (second edition).

Diane Trippett, M.S., R.D., Clinical Nutrition Manager of the Dietetics Department of Children's Hospital of Michigan, Detroit, Michigan.

"Eating Disorders" reviewed by David Rosen, M.D., M.P.H., C.S. Mott Children's Hospital, A. Alfred Taubman Health Care Center, Ann Arbor, Michigan.

"Dental Health" written by Craig C. Spangler, D.D.S., Bloomfield Hills, Michigan.

Chapter 5

TEENS AND MENTAL ILLNESS

Depressive Illnesses

Depression affects over 15 million adult Americans each year, yet only about one-third of those affected get treatment. Ironically, among all psychiatric illnesses—which is what depression is—depression is among the most responsive to treatment. Given the huge rise in teen suicide rates over the last 25 years, families need to know about depressive illnesses just as they know about other illnesses and health factors that affect teens. While depression has a genetic component, it is often triggered by situations and stresses that people perceive as hopeless.

Serious depression, usually called *clinical depression*, is not something for adults or teens to treat alone. At the very least, teens don't have the time to stop their lives—to suffer at home, miss school, and endure the whole-body pain that comes with depression—to be depressed. At the worst, untreated depression can lead to suicide.

Recognizing Depression

Sorting out the signs of depression, as opposed to the normal mood swings of adolescence, is hard. Often times, adults see the signs of depression as a phase their teen is going through. Some people mistakenly believe that dealing with depression is a matter of will, something a person could "snap out of" if they "just wanted to." Alcohol and drug abuse greatly complicate matters.

Many teens see depression as a weakness and therefore something to hide. Most teens will have trouble, especially if they are depressed, connecting their emotional state to their behavior. That helps explains why poor school performance is often the first indicator of a more serious problem. In general, teens are better at saying how they feel, while adults are better observers of their teen's behavior. Before you read about the signs of depression, note two mandates that every adult should follow regarding depression.

- In any instance where you think your teen may be suffering from depression, seek a psychiatrist or psychologist who is experienced in working with depressed adolescents.
- Seek professional help immediately, regardless of whether or not you think your teen is depressed, if your teen talks about wanting to die or wishing that he or she was dead.

Signs of Depression

Seek professional help for your teen if you notice five or more of the following symptoms for two weeks or longer.

- Lowered mood most of the day and nearly every day, or unexplained hyperactivity.
- Uncharacteristic lack of interest in daily activities, especially school, friendships, hobbies, and outside interests.
- Major changes in weight or appetite.
- Sleeping too little or too much.

- Feeling worthless, useless, or excessively guilty.
- Problems concentrating, thinking, or making decisions.
- Recurrent thoughts or statements about death or dying.

Bipolar Disorder

Bipolar disorder (formerly called manic-depression) is the most severe form of depression, and usually begins in adolescence or early adulthood. One way to think about this illness is in terms of a cycle or wave of moods. At the bottom of the wave is depression. The middle of the wave is normal. Higher up, there is mild mania, a time of more energy, ideas, and sometimes more sex drive. At the crest of the wave is mania, a period marked by rocketing energy, overflowing thoughts and emotions, and often serious behavior problems and periods of marked poor judgment.

For many people suffering from Bipolar Disorder, life is a roller coaster that either won't start or starts going too fast, with normal periods sandwiched between. Luckily, there are many effective treatments for Bipolar Disorder.

Complicating Factors

As with depression, the family's greatest barrier in getting an accurate diagnosis of Bipolar Disorder may be denial that there *is* a problem. Adding to that may be alcohol and/or drug use by the teen.

Adults with mental health issues are 2.7 times more likely to have an alcohol or other substance abuse problem than other people in the population. Adults with alcohol or drug problems are 4.5 times more likely to have some sort of underlying mental health problem. To complicate matters just a little more, "self-medication" with alcohol and drugs is fairly typical of people with Bipolar Disorder. Drugs like cocaine are often used as a means to fight depression; alcohol is often used to fight periods of mania or as short-term relief against depression. Self-medication not only *doesn't* work, it actually hides the symptoms of depression or Bipolar Disorder, and can make effective treatment of either illness almost impossible.

Any treatment for depression or Bipolar Disorder needs to include a close look at *any* alcohol or drug use. All morality aside, alcohol and drugs—especially if used while taking medication for either illness—complicate an already difficult medical problem and throw a monkey wrench into any medical or therapeutic solution to the problem. If your teen is experiencing problems with depression, he or she needs you to get very serious about any alcohol or drug use.

New Hope for Prevention

In his widely respected book, *Emotional Intelligence*, author Daniel Goleman reports on new research that shows it may be possible to head off or decrease the severity of depression in young people. These studies pinpoint two areas that can lead youth into a downward spiral of negative thought patterns. First, poor relationship skills can create a pattern of isolation in which sadness and negative inner feelings don't get expressed or resolved. As the child or teen becomes more cut off from others, those negative feelings increase. Second, a pessimistic response to life's failures, rejections, and losses also leads to increasing sadness, poor self-esteem, and isolation from family and friends.

In one study, mildly depressed students attended special classes where they learned to identify and challenge these habits of thought, and were taught new social skills. When compared with a similar group that did not receive the instruction, the students who attended the special classes were found to be more likely to have recovered from their mild depression, and less likely to develop severe depression later on.

This research does not contradict the idea that the factors that put people at risk for severe depression are largely genetic and biological. What it does suggest is that it may be possible for children and teens to learn skills and habits of mind that may lessen their risk of actually falling into a severe depression. The key is for family members or other perceptive people in a teen's life to recognize symptoms of the problem early and take the right steps.

Teen Suicide

This year, about 10,000 teens will commit suicide. Another 400,000 teens will make suicide attempts. Over one million teens will slide in and out of despair and hopelessness so severe that their thoughts turn to suicide.

Suicide is the third leading cause of death among teens ages fifteen to nineteen, trailing only traffic accidents and homi-cide. Compared to 25 years ago, teen suicides are up some 300 percent. Adolescent girls attempt suicide more often than adolescent boys—perhaps as much as eight times more often—but male suicide attempts are more violent and result in death more often.

For most teens, the wish to die is less powerful than the message a suicide attempt sends to parents and loved ones. Unfortunately, risking one's life to send a message puts teen suicide in a different category than any other issue affecting teens, parents, and families. "It's a cry for help" used to be the buzz phrase for suicide attempts. While that does explain some suicide attempts, adults need to know that teen suicide attempts fall into dozens of categories.

Some teens develop suicidal thoughts in response to the death of a loved one or friend. Some teens see suicide as the only answer to unbearable pain and suffering in their lives. Rejection in an intimate relationship or the denial of a longed-for relationship, a perceived or real public humiliation, or failure to achieve an expected goal—things adults may see as merely troublesome or even trivial in the lives of their child—are often extremely traumatic to a teen. Perfectionists are particularly vulnerable. Some teens never make a single suicide attempt, but live their lives in chronic alienation from their families and society, constantly pursuing high-risk behaviors such as alcohol and drug use, unprotected sex, and thrill-seeking suicidal games.

Here are some possible triggering events that may lead a teen to think of and/or attempt suicide.

- Break up of a significant relationship with a girlfriend or boyfriend.
- Divorce in the family.
- Recent loss of a loved one or friend.
- Recent failure to reach a much-desired goal, or loss of a job.

Warning Signs of Suicidal Intent

The majority of suicidal teens suffer from depression. Parents should call a doctor, psychiatrist, or the local hospital for a counseling referral if their teen begins to show the following signs of depression—especially if they are *uncharacteristic* of their son's or daughter's usual personality. Signs may include extended withdrawal from school or social activities (especially daily family interaction), lack of concern for appearance, falling or failing grades, markedly increased irritability and intolerance, crying easily or for no apparent reason, physical fighting at home or school, increased alcohol or drug use.

Seek professional help *immediately* if your teen begins to use expressions such as "I can't take it anymore," or "I want to die," or talks about joining someone who is already dead. Other *serious* signs of depression might be any of the following, or similar behaviors.

- Giving a note to a friend to give to a family member "in a couple of days."
- Giving away valued objects.
- Making plans to donate body.
- Collecting pills or other medications.
- Buying a gun.

Tips for Preventing Suicide

- *Do not* leave a potentially suicidal teen alone.
- *Do not* take any mention of suicide or death lightly.
- *Do* get involved, and stay involved.
- *Do* show your care and concern in every way you can.
- *Do not* play amateur psychologist— seek professional help.
- Call your local hospital or crisis center.
- Contact your school. Schools often have a crisis counselor.
- Contact a favorite teacher or other favorite adult in your teen's life.
- *Do* use every resource you can think of to help your child—you may save a life.

"Depressive Illnesses" *adapted from* "Mood Disorders in Childhood and Adolescence—Part I," The Harvard Mental Health Letter, *Volume 10, Number 5, November 1993, and* "Recognizing Depression Key to Treatment," The Menninger Letter, *January 1996.*

Contributions to and review of entire chapter by:

Pam Farlow-Wolgast, M.A., L.L.P., L.P.C., C.S.W., Staff Training and Development Coordinator, Common Ground, Pontiac, Michigan.

Betty Tableman, M.P.A., Director, Prevention Services, Michigan Department of Community Health, Lansing, Michigan.

Joel L. Young, M.D., Medical Director, Psychiatric Evaluation and Referral Center, Crittenton Hospital, Rochester, Michigan.

Chapter 6

A STUDY ON TEEN SUBSTANCE ABUSE

Monitoring the Future

We owe a deep debt of gratitude to Dr. Lloyd D. Johnston and his colleagues at The University of Michigan, Survey Research Center in Ann Arbor, Michigan, for the all-important information you are about to read. Dr. Johnston, a social research psychologist, is an internationally recognized expert in drug use among teens, and is the principal investigator of the 22-year-old Monitoring the Future *study. We also extend our special thanks to those professionals who reviewed our work, and to the many other researchers, writers, and practitioners in the field of substance abuse prevention whose material we have studied.*

This chapter provides up-to-date statistics on the use of substances by teens from the *1996 Monitoring the Future* study. Chapter 7, "Preventing Teen Substance Abuse," details how parents and families can help teens avoid substance abuse. Chapter 8, "Teens and the Drugs They Use" contains facts about substances and their effects on teens. Chapter 9, "Teens Who Use Drugs," carefully spells out the consequences of teen substance abuse. Chapter 9 also includes tips on recognizing the problem and what to seek help. "Appendix C" contains a table of 1996 Michigan laws on substances, and a section entitled, "The Law and Adults."

1996 Study Results

Adults need to know the facts about drug use among teens. These figures are the latest from the *Monitoring the Future* study, a series of annual surveys of some 49,000 students in over 435 public and private secondary schools nationwide.

- 24 percent of eighth graders used an illegal drug in the last year, up from 11 percent in 1991.
- 38 percent of tenth graders used an illegal drug in the last year, up from 21 percent in 1991.
- 40 percent of twelfth graders used an illegal drug in the last year, up from 29 percent in 1991.

Substance abuse among teens concerns all responsible people around the world. Drug use among teens continues to rise from levels of use reported during the late 1980's. Attitudes and beliefs about the dangers and consequences of drug use continue to soften among teens—a fact that is largely responsible for the upward turn in drug use.

Teens today know less about drugs and the dangers of drug use than the generation of teens before them. Since the Gulf War in 1991, anti-drug messages on television and from public figures have dropped significantly. As the earlier drug epidemic has subsided, younger children have had fewer opportunities to learn through informal means about the dangers of drugs. Previous groups of young children learned by observing bad outcomes of drug abuse by other young people around them. In addition, says Johnston, a number of groups in the recording industry—particularly rap, grunge, and rock musicians—began to send pro-drug messages through their lyrics, album and song titles, and personal behavior on stage and off. Thus, in addition to hearing fewer cautions about drugs, teens have increasingly heard some people sing their praises. All of these factors contribute to what Dr. Johnston calls "generational forgetting." What is the result of this generational forgetting? A steady rise in drug use among teens over the last six years, and a *dramatic* rise in marijuana use among teens.

Monitoring Tobacco

Tobacco use is also up for teens of all ages. Over the past year (between 1995 and 1996), the percentage of students reporting any cigarette smoking in the thirty days prior to the survey rose by about 10 percent among both eighth- and tenth-graders. Over the past five years (1991-96), the proportion of kids reporting smoking in the prior thirty days has risen by nearly one-half among the eighth-graders (from 14 percent to 21 percent) and tenth-graders (from 21 percent to 30 percent). Among twelfth-graders, the proportional increases have been lower, but still appreciable.

In summary, in 1996, current smoking rates were 21 percent among eighth-graders (13-14 years old), 30 percent among tenth-graders (15-16 years old), and 34 percent among twelfth-graders (17-18 years old). These rates are impressively high, especially when compared to the fact that about 25 percent of all adults are classified as current smokers according to the National Health Interview Survey.

Aside from the well-known risks of long-term smoking, experts like Johnston believe that cigarette smoking is strongly tied to smoking marijuana. Smoking cigarettes usually comes before smoking marijuana—teaching teens how to take smoke into their lungs for a drug-induced effect. Teens who smoke already know how to get high when it comes to smoking marijuana. Johnston and others believe that the rise in cigarette smoking among teens may well have contributed to the rise in marijuana use.

Monitoring Marijuana

The 1996 study found that marijuana use is leading the way in the rise of drug use among teens. Again, the facts tell the first part of the story. The following figures reflect reported marijuana use in the previous twelve months.

- Marijuana use among eighth-graders tripled from 6 percent in 1991 to 18 percent in 1996.
- Marijuana use among tenth-graders increased from a low of 15 percent in 1992 to more than double that number, 34 percent, in 1996.
- Marijuana use among twelfth-graders increased from a low of 22 percent in 1992 to 36 percent in 1996.

Of particular concern to Johnston is the continuing rise in *daily* marijuana use. The study reported the following increases for all three grade levels studied. Nearly 5 percent of high school students smoke marijuana on a daily basis; 3.3 percent of tenth-graders used marijuana on a daily basis; and 1.5 percent of eighth-graders use the drug *every day*.

The rapid rise in the number of teens using marijuana points to a rise in the pool of teens who are willing to consider using other drugs, and helps explain the increase in use of other illegal drugs besides marijuana. Furthermore, the proportional increases have been even greater for the younger children.

While marijuana has shown the most dramatic rise in use among teens, a number of other drugs also show an increase between 1991 and 1996. Hallucinogens (primarily LSD), inhalants, stimulants, barbiturates, cocaine, and crack cocaine all showed a gradual upturn in the 1996 study.

Monitoring Inhalants

"One of the brighter parts of the story involves the use of inhalants by young people," notes Dr. Johnston. (Inhalants encompass a broad class of volatile substances such as glues, solvents, butane, and nitrous oxide. Their use tends to be highest among younger teens.) "After four years of steady increase in inhalant use by young people, we are seeing a leveling and perhaps the beginning of a reversal in 1996." The proportion of eighth-, tenth- and twelfth-graders reporting any inhalant use in the prior twelve months is 12 percent, 10 percent, and 8 percent, respectively, in 1996.

"We believe we know something about why this turnaround has occurred," Johnston continues. "We are seeing in the 1996 results a sharp increase in the proportions of students indicating that they view inhalant use as dangerous.

After this study called attention to the magnitude of the inhalant problem a few years ago, there were various efforts undertaken to educate youngsters to the dangers of this class of drugs, including a public service advertising initiative by the Partnership for a Drug Free America. The changes in students beliefs about the dangers of inhalant use suggest that the various efforts are working: disapproval of inhalant use has begun to rise."

Monitoring Alcohol

American teens drink often and in large quantities. Although there is no great change in the reported use of alcohol in 1996, all three grades surveyed showed a general rise in use. For example, 16 percent of eighth-graders reported having five or more drinks in a row during the previous two-week period. The reported rates rise as teens get older. Some 25 percent of tenth-graders reported having more than five or more drinks in a row during a two week period. For twelfth-graders, the figure remained at 30 percent (from 1995). Self-reported drunkenness by twelfth-graders increased somewhat in 1996.

Education and Prevention

Experts like Dr. Lloyd D. Johnston are the first to note that drug use among teens today is not nearly as high as it was during the peak years in the late 1970's. Johnston is also a strong advocate of the power of families, communities, and society as a whole to reduce drug use among teens. "Each new generation needs to learn the same lessons about drugs if they are going to be protected from them," says Johnston. In short, the answer to "generational forgetting" is education and prevention. The information that follows is designed to give families the tools they need to work with their teen to prevent or stop substance use.

Reviewed by Joyce Buchanan, Administrative Assistant to Dr. Lloyd D. Johnston, The University of Michigan "Monitoring the Future" *study, Survey Research Center, Ann Arbor, Michigan.*

Chapter 7

PREVENTING TEEN SUBSTANCE ABUSE

A Family Model

Many families today *are* working with their teen to prevent drug use, whether the drug is nicotine in cigarettes, marijuana, alcohol, inhalants, or any other kind of drug. The model these families are using is inclusive: No drug use of any kind is acceptable. This model involves the teen in the reasoning and decision-making process and focuses on clear-cut rules and consequences. The line these adults have decided to walk goes beyond simply forbidding drug use with words and threats, to knowing the realities of drug use among teens, the temptations teens face, and a willingness to have a relationship with their teen that makes "no drug use" work for both the families and their teen.

Here are three reasons an adult can use as the basis to prohibit all drug use.

- *Drugs are dangerous.* What *is* known about drug use among teens points to disaster, whether the result is a life-long addiction to cigarettes or an early death in an alcohol-related traffic accident. There is absolutely *no* evidence to show that drug use in teens is not dangerous, and not getting more dangerous. A fight when high or drunk could lead to a shooting; having sex in the same condition could lead to pregnancy or sexually transmitted disease.
- *Drug use is illegal.* The chart in "Appendix C" details Michigan laws about drug use. Adults need to know

these laws and lean on these laws when setting rules about drug use with their teen. Quoting laws might seem hypocritical to some people, or at least not a very sound argument, but the facts are the facts. At the very least, teens need to know that parents or other adults may be held responsible for their teen's drug or alcohol use, and for the teen's actions while under the influence of drugs. Parents, not teens, are the ones who bear the burden of late night trips to the local jail, dealing with the police, the courts, the schools, and worst of all, the funeral expenses.

- *Drug use doesn't mix with our family values, school, sports, and the other activities of a teen.* This is a tough time to grow up as a teen. Compared to 25 or 30 years ago, today's teen faces increased risks for all manner of life-threatening situations, whether that be suicide, teen pregnancy, contracting HIV, or being involved in a homicide. At the very least, teens need to know that drug use makes doing well in school harder, will affect their emotional life, and make it harder to make and keep quality friends. Teens today need every break they can get to protect their health and potential for success.

Teens Saying No to Drugs

There is more involved in preventing drug use than just setting rules. Your teen needs a strong sense of self-esteem, along with the social skills necessary to withstand peer pressure to participate in substance abuse and other risky behaviors. Your teen needs to know that he or she is loved and valued as a person.

As with any issue involving your teen, planning and spending time with your teen on a daily basis is the key to lasting success. Your son or daughter needs to see how the rules you have set work with the experiences they have outside of the home, at school, and with friends. Your son or daughter needs to know the consequences of breaking rules, of course, but it is probably more important for him or her to know that *you are aware* of the drug use in your community and the fact that he or she will be offered drugs and will have the opportunity to use drugs.

Families need to give their teen every possible, simple way to refuse drugs. You need to be willing to work with your teen on easy, no-nonsense ways to say no to drugs. In most cases, this means letting your teen off the hook, and putting yourself in the role as the heavy. A teen who says "I made a deal with my family not to use drugs" faces a fewer questions than a teen left facing their peers alone. Likewise, a simple, short answer for saying no to drugs holds up better to follow-up questions. "Look, what can I say, I made a deal with my family," is a simple, straightforward response—one that can be followed by a another, equally simple response. "Don't

you get it? A deal's a deal, and I'm keeping my end of the bargain."

Adults who expect their teens not to use drugs have to also be willing to listen to their teen talk about drug use around them. Adults even need to be willing to accept some small lapse in the rules—a beer at a party, a hit off a joint—in exchange for their teen's willingness to talk about the situation. A two-way street is just that. The more your teen is willing to talk with you about drugs, the better the chance that your teen will stay off drugs.

Reviewed by:

Katherine Miller, M.A., Prevention Section Chief, Office of Substance Abuse Services, Michigan Department of Community Health, Lansing, Michigan.

Pat Morgan, R.N., M.S., Consultant for School Health Programs, School Health Unit, Michigan Department of Community Health, Lansing, Michigan.

Andrea Poniers, M.S.S.W., Public Health Consultant, Tobacco Section, Center for Health Promotion, Chronic Disease Prevention, Michigan Department of Community Health, Lansing, Michigan.

Donald B. Sweeney, M.A., Chief, School Health Unit, Michigan Department of Community Health, Lansing, Michigan.

Betty Tableman, M.P.A., Director, Prevention Services, Michigan Department of Community Health, Lansing, Michigan.

Chapter 8

TEENS AND THE DRUGS THEY USE

Teens and Tobacco

There are two vital issues adults need to face about teen tobacco use. First, if you do not use tobacco, you can't assume your teen will follow suit. Second, if you do use tobacco, your teen is statistically more likely to also use tobacco. If you are a tobacco user, be straightforward with your teen about your own use. Point out the reasons you started using tobacco and be prepared to admit that you are addicted to nicotine. If you have smoked in the past but quit, talk with your teen about the addictive nature of tobacco and how hard it was to quit.

If you don't use tobacco, talk about how hard it was to resist starting when you were a teen. Many people find it easiest to talk about the short-term effects of tobacco use first—the high cost, smelly clothes, bad breath, and yellowing teeth. You may wish to discuss the following facts as well.

- Tobacco use is considered a gateway drug to other drug use.
- Nicotine found in tobacco is a highly addictive drug. Teens who have smoked or chewed for only a short time have as much trouble quitting as long-time tobacco users. It's much better never to start a tobacco habit.
- Tobacco use immediately affects the user's lung capacity, especially in terms of athletics.
- Tobacco users have more coughs and illnesses than non-users.
- Most people do not use tobacco.

- Tobacco use is becoming much less socially acceptable, at school, in the workplace, and in public places.

The next step for families is to know—and talk about—the long-term effects of tobacco use. Talking about lung cancer, throat cancer, heart attacks, or strokes may have some influence on your teen. Most people find that they need to break the topic down into information that shows how tobacco use leads to illness.

- Nicotine increases blood pressure, raises the heart rate, and causes blood vessels to constrict and become narrower.
- Carbon monoxide in cigarette smoke interferes with oxygen delivery to the blood, steals oxygen's place on red blood cells, and decreases oxygen in the body and heart. Blood in the body becomes thicker as a result.

Smoking causes heart disease, lung cancer, and emphysema. There are no clearer facts than those, and it says so on every pack of cigarettes. The Centers for Disease Control's "Guidelines for School Health Programs to Prevent Tobacco Use and Addiction" (*Morbidity and Mortality Weekly Report*, February 25, 1994) states the following facts.

Recent estimates suggest that cigarette smoking causes more than 400,000 premature deaths annually and 5 million years of potential life lost. . . . Tobacco use is addictive and is responsible for more than one of every five deaths in the United States. However, many children and adolescents do not understand the nature of tobacco addiction and are unaware of, or underestimate, the important health consequences of tobacco use. On average, more than 3,000 young people, most of them children and teenagers, begin smoking each day in the United States. Approximately 82 percent of adults ages thirty to thirty-nine years who ever smoked daily tried their first cigarette before eighteen years of age.

Cigarette use is the most avoidable cause of death in the United States. Whether you smoke or not, you can raise a teen who does not. You have every right to work out rules about tobacco use with your teen to keep your teen tobacco free.

In describing findings from the University of Michigan *1996 Monitoring the Future* study, Dr. Lloyd Johnston concludes, "Because young people tend to carry the smoking habits they develop in adolescence into adulthood, the substantial and continuing increases in teen smoking bode ill for the eventual longevity and health of this generation of American young people. Hundreds of thousands of children from each graduating class are likely to suffer appalling diseases, and to die prematurely, as a result of the smoking habits they are developing in childhood and adolescence."

Teens and Alcohol

Drinking and driving is *the* leading cause of death among teens. Unfortunately,

alcohol use and abuse is a problem that affects our whole society. A recent Cornell University study looked at 224 hours of prime-time TV programs (not ads). Researchers took note of all the examples of eating and drinking during prime-time programs. Drinking alcohol and eating snacks were the most commonly shown food scenes.

Alcohol consumption is a massive complex of issues that, on the one hand, seems to point toward socializing, fun, and good times. On the other hand, it points toward violent deaths, shattered lives, and potential lost. Recovering alcoholics talk about lives "performed" on the stage, under the lights of a play best called "Death on the Installment Plan."

Like their elders, American teens drink at a high rate. Children as young as eight and nine list alcohol as a problem in *their* lives, whether the problem is caused by the drinking done by other people in their lives, or by their own drinking.

You can drink moderately yourself and raise a teen who does not drink. Your role as a parent and adult supports such a stance. The law, and the often the fatal mistakes teens make while drunk or drinking, support such a stance. There is nothing hypocritical about telling your teen that alcohol is something that adults can enjoy—and something that he or she might enjoy as an adult—but is simply not allowed now. Ask yourself, "What would you tell a fourteen-year-old who wants to drive the family car?"

If you drink, explain to your teen why you drink, and take some time to look at your own drinking habits. As with most behavior, teens are often better observers then they are listeners. Your drinking habits will definitely influence your teen. "What you do speaks so loudly, I cannot hear what you say," holds true.

Alcoholism in Your Family

Finally, let your teen know if there is a history of alcoholism in your family. No amount of shame or pride should keep you from being straightforward about his or her family history. Many, many young lives would be saved the slow death of alcoholism or pain of recovering from alcohol by knowing at an early age that alcohol may not be something they can handle in even small amounts—because of the genetic risk in your family. If parental alcoholism is also a factor in your home, you may wish to contact the National Association for Children of Alcoholics (NACoA), in Rockville, Maryland for additional help for your teen (telephone 301-468-0985).

In addition to hearing where your family stands on alcohol, your teen needs to know the basic facts about alcohol, the facts that other teens usually don't know, and facts that special interest groups spend millions to distort and glamorize.

- Alcohol is a drug. Specifically, alcohol is a *depressant.*
- Alcohol slows body functions, coordination, and the ability to think and react.
- Alcohol affects everyone differently, but, in general, body weight and the amount of alcohol consumed over time are the two most important factors.

- Alcohol affects judgment and lowers inhibitions. Teens who are drinking or drunk do things they would not ordinarily do. Behaviors range from becoming upset emotionally, fighting, using other drugs, participating in unplanned sexual activity—including unsafe sex—to drinking and driving.
- Alcohol generally lowers sexual inhibitions, but actually also lowers sexual performance and enjoyment.

Teens should also know that drinking very large amounts of alcohol over a short period of time, say a tumbler full of hard liquor, can cause sudden death. Finally, alcoholic beverages should never be confused with poisonous products that contain alcohol. Rubbing alcohol, for example, is not an alcoholic beverage and may be fatal if swallowed.

As with all discussions regarding drugs, families need to set clear expectations for behavior, clear rules, and clear consequences for breaking the rules, without making drinking seem appealing as something to do because it is forbidden.

Teens and Marijuana

For many adults, their own past marijuana use is a barrier to talking with their teen about marijuana today. The choices you made when you were young are just that—choices made in the past. As a parent and as an adult you need to address this issue in the present tense, and focus on the facts about marijuana today, your family values today, and what the world is like for teens today. Consider the following basic facts about marijuana.

- Marijuana today has much higher level of THC (the chemical that produces the high) than before, especially compared to marijuana available in the 1960s.
- Faulty judgment while using marijuana puts teens at increased risks for automobile accidents, unplanned and unsafe sexual practices, drowning, falls, and even suicide.
- Marijuana use may slow sexual development.
- Teens who smoke pot are at increased risk for cancer. One study found that one marijuana cigarette produced the same lung damage as five tobacco cigarettes.
- Teens who smoke marijuana are more likely to smoke cigarettes, use other drugs, and drink alcohol.

Most teens—and most adults—are familiar with marijuana. The general softening stance of many adults, teens, and society as a whole has been well documented. The huge rise in marijuana use among teens is well documented. Few people, however, are willing to confront the facts: Your teen may already be getting high; your teen is being or will be offered the chance to get high and to use other drugs. Parents need to somehow marry those facts—the realities for teens—with what they really want for their son or daughter. Take a stand today, if only to talk to your teen about the facts of marijuana use presented above.

Teens and Inhalants

Inhalants are readily available and inexpensive. Aerosol sprays, gasoline, spray paint, nail polish remover, glue, paint

---

Effects of Inhalants
Short-term
- Appearing intoxicated.
- Chemical-smelling breath.
- Dazed or dizzy appearance.
- Slurred speech.
- Excitability.

Long-term
- A decrease in appetite.
- Runny nose or nose bleeds.
- Rashes around the mouth or nose.
- Poor memory.
- Loss of coordination.
- Hand tremors
- Chronic coughing

---

thinner, and any number of other materials can be used as inhalants. The inhalant is usually sprayed or poured onto a rag or into a paper bag and the fumes inhaled through the mouth and nose. Sounds crazy doesn't it? The fact is that using inhalants is a very dangerous practice and can be fatal.

- Inhaled fumes are absorbed into the bloodstream and passed to organs within seconds.
- Inhalants cause the user to grow tolerant to the effects of the high, resulting in a need to use more and more inhalant material over time.
- Inhalants may cause irregular heartbeat and lead to sudden death, result in lack of coordination, hearing and memory loss, and mental illness, and damage the brain, kidneys, heart, and bone marrow.

Inhalants are most commonly used by younger teens—kids in the sixth through ninth grades. Aside from the sheer danger of the practice, researchers believe that there is a strong connection between learning to get high on inhalants and using other drugs later on. The first step for families is to help younger teens understand that "sniffing" is drug use, and has serious consequences.

Reviewed by:

Katherine Miller, M.A., Prevention Section Chief, Office of Substance Abuse Services, Michigan Department of Community Health, Lansing, Michigan.

James Moore, Program Director and Assistant Executive Director, American Lung Association, Lansing, Michigan.

Pat Morgan, R.N., M.S., Consultant for School Health Programs, School Health Unit, Michigan Department of Community Health, Lansing, Michigan.

Andrea Poniers, M.S.S.W., Public Health Consultant, Tobacco Section, Center for Health Promotion, Chronic Disease Prevention, Michigan Department of Community Health, Lansing, Michigan.

Donald B. Sweeney, M.A., Chief, School Health Unit, Michigan Department of Community Health, Lansing, Michigan.

Betty Tableman, M.P.A., Director, Prevention Services, Michigan Department of Community Health, Lansing, Michigan.

Sis Wenger, M.A., Executive Director of the National Association of Children of Alcoholics (NACOA), Rockville, Maryland.

Chapter 9

TEENS WHO USE DRUGS

Facing the Problem

One of the grander myths about the American family is that a family solves its own problems, quietly and effectively. A family is strong and supportive—a last sanctuary for any problem or crisis. When it comes to helping a teen stop using drugs, many families try to promote this myth of the American family and hide the problem, or go just the opposite route and find blame for the problem in every aspect of society *except* their own family and their teen. Getting a teen off drugs and *keeping* that teen off drugs—regardless of the drug—is tough, grueling, and often painful work.

A family needs to admit and accept their teen's drug use, reserve blame, and look forward with the single, sole-minded task of getting their teen off drugs. Neither dropping a teen off at a hospital or rehabilitation center and hoping for the best, or denying the problem—simply ignoring the drug use or taking blame for the problem—works. The figures and statistics about recovery from drug or alcohol abuse are grim. Caring adults can either be involved on the upside to recovery or the downside to continued use. Those are the same options available for a teen using drugs.

Recognizing the Problem

The first step for families is to recognize that there *is* a problem. For better or worse, there are any number of objective factors that point toward drug use. For example, traffic tickets for driving under the influence of alcohol are a very good indicator of alcohol abuse. Low grades, absenteeism, withdrawal from family activities, unexplained injuries or accidents can also be objective indicators of a drug problem. However, those indicators are often more complex than answering a simple question. Where is my teen spending his or her time, and what is he or she doing during that time? It takes time to get drugs, use drugs, and then return home. Another simple way to ask the same question is, "Where is my teen spending his or her energy?" The fewer answers you have to the questions above, the more you need to know. It is not normal for a teen to be out all night, sleep during the day, and then be unexpectedly frantic to go out the next night. When you think about drugs and your teen, think objectively and coolly.

Denial

Most people with a drug problem will deny it. Generally, the greater the problem, the greater the denial. For this reason, prying facts about drug use out teens is usually not very productive. Most people have more success presenting their teen with a list of objective behaviors that point to a problem that they want to solve with their teen. Sometimes the problem is something else. Give your teen a break. Stick to facts, and ask your teen to respond. If you are uncomfortable with such a confrontation, contact a local crisis center or community health agency and ask what they think about your observations and how you might proceed. There may be an underlying depressive illness causing your teen to seek "self-medication." A crisis center professional may be able to help you sort out facts, identify the problem, consider possible solutions, and then decide on what to do next.

Getting Help

The outcome of your discussion or discussions with your teen may lead you to seek professional help. For many people, it is tempting to seek psychological help for their teen. If you decide to go this route, make sure that the counselor or therapist knows that you are very concerned about your teen's drug use. Again, a few simple rules apply. It is difficult—some say impossible—to treat an active drug user. Many therapists will not diagnose or treat a teen until the drug use has stopped for at least a few months. Don't allow anyone who downplays drug use to treat your teen. The risk to your teen is too great. There is no psychological or medical solution that works in conjunction with continued drug abuse.

Many families seek a more complete answer to their teen's drug use at a hospital or drug treatment center. You should know that more and more hospitals and treatment centers are treating drug use on an out-patient basis. Hospitalization is increasingly being reserved for emergencies and detoxification. Cost is certainly a factor, but more important reasons for out-patient treatment are recent study results about the effectiveness of treating drug use.

Studies show that the number of hours a *patient* spent learning about their drug problem and recovery were the most significant factors in recovery. In other words, keeping a patient physically away from drugs is less important than the patient learning about their problem and how to recover. Of course, there are still many private institutions that provide in-patient care over a period of weeks or even months.

Choosing a treatment plan for your teen can be confusing. Treatment centers range in cost and amenities from the Salvation Army to the Betty Ford Clinic. Fortunately, your own community will probably have a fairly wide range of treatment centers. Talking with a trained drug and alcohol counselor, your religious leader, your doctor, or any adult you are comfortable with and trust will usually yield a solution that fits the problem your teen has. Depending on your teen's situation and condition, you may want to discuss treatment options with him or her. Your teen is not the first person who has had a drug problem.

Support for Your Teen

Drug use and alcoholism—whether or not you wish to call either a disease—are both, in part, defined by relapse, returning to abuse. Few people seek help for their own problem, fewer people are drug free one year after treatment, and very, very, few people are drug free for the rest of their lives. It is no surprise then, that the most effective treatment programs tend to focus on one day at time. The other general trend in treatment and recovery programs is toward individual responsibility—for behavior toward one's self and others—and developing a work ethic that includes practical as well as spiritual matters. At the core, good treatment centers realize the need to change how a person thinks about his or her drug use, whether that means facing the objective facts of how their use affected them, or challenging how the user thinks about drug use.

Effective treatment centers always involve the family of the patient. Families need to know what they can do to help, but probably more important, *families need to show up for their teen*. Recovery is frightening and difficult for anyone, but many families are often blind to the power of the simplest kinds of help they can provide. Showing up for family sessions, talking with counselors, and listening to your teen don't require much effort, but often have a striking effect on the person in recovery.

Finally, you need to have hope and strength that their teen will get help. Any drug user in recovery will tell you that each single day of recovery is hard won and a blessing. Don't give up on your teen. A day clean and sober, whether that is day one or many, many days later, is the only real way to a useful and productive life for most drug users.

Reviewed by:

Joyce Buchanan, Administrative Assistant to Dr. Lloyd D. Johnston, The University of Michigan "Monitoring the Future" Study, Survey Research Center, Ann Arbor, Michigan.

Detective Ron Halcrow of the Birmingham Police Department, Birmingham, Michigan.

The Michigan Department of State Police: Sergeant Joseph Hanley of the Special Operations Division, Traffic Services Division; Lt. Dan Smith of the Traffic Services Division; and Phyllis Good, Supervisor of the Narcotics and Dangerous Drugs Unit, East Lansing Laboratory, East Lansing, Michigan.

Katherine Miller, Prevention Section Chief, Office of Substance Abuse Services, Michigan Department of Community Health, Lansing, Michigan.

James Moore, Program Manager and Assistant Executive Director, American Lung Association, - Lansing, Michigan.

Pat Morgan, Consultant for School Health Programs, School Health Unit, Michigan Department of Community Health, Lansing, Michigan.

Andrea Poniers, Public Health Consultant, Tobacco Section, Center for Health Promotion, Chronic Disease Prevention, Michigan Department of Community Health, Lansing, Michigan.

Donald B. Sweeney, M.A., Chief, School Health Unit, Michigan Department of Community Health, Lansing, Michigan.

Sis Wenger, Executive Director of the National Association of Children of Alcoholics (NACOA), Rockville, Maryland.

Chapter 10

TEENS AND SEXUALITY

Educating Your Teen

There is good news for adults when it comes to talking with their teen about sex: The process began when you first held your child as an infant—and it continued on a daily basis as your son or daughter observed your attitudes and behaviors toward sex and the human body. Hopefully, you've been fielding questions about sex as a normal part of parenting, especially in the preteen years from 9 to 13 when sex is a distant consideration. Even if you've never said a word about sex (which is not an excuse to remain silent any longer!), your actions, attitudes, and your own relationships are a framework for more direct discussions about sex with your teen.

If you make sex education an ongoing process—something normal for you to discuss—you can save yourself and your teen from the awkward, one-time, big-deal conversation about sex. You may remember this talk yourself; one that started, "We need to talk, woman to woman" or "Son, let's have a talk."

Young children ask lots of questions, but remember, your answers should be appropriate to their ages. At five or six years of age, most children in our culture don't care about the mechanics of sexual behavior, and many would be confused by the details. Your attitudes and feelings about what is right or wrong, however, are important to communicate early. Remember, how we relate to members of the opposite sex is more than just a matter of sexual intercourse.

The next bit of good news is that nine out of ten teens say they want to learn about sex from their parents. Unfortunately, fewer than one teen in ten can actually rely on his or her family for the information they need to know about sex.

Finally, there has never before been as strong a public, political, and social mandate for families to educate their children about sex. Consider the facts.

- 74 percent of today's teens—boys *and* girls—will have engaged in sex before they graduate from high school.
- There are over 1 million teen pregnancies a year in the United States.
- To date, there is no cure for HIV/-AIDS.

Caring adults today cannot ignore their important role in sex education. As an adult with a teenager, you have to decide what your teen needs to know about sex, and how to talk about sex to your teen.

Families as Teachers

One reason people give for not talking about sex is the fear that talking about sex somehow encourages sexual activity or implies giving permission to have sex. Research has clearly shown that there is absolutely no connection between sex education—in the home or at school—and increased sexual activity. None. What researchers *do* find is a connection between a lack of sex education and teen pregnancies. Despite what some adults and many teens think, statistics show that young people today are just as ignorant about sex as the generations of teens that came before them.

One of your most important roles as a parent is to help your teen develop healthy sexual attitudes and behaviors. Your values and your attitudes are the most important part of the process. You may wish, however, to think of your role as having other, equally important, parts.

- *Face the facts about the world your teen lives in*—Talk to a friend, call your teen's school, or visit your public library. Find out for yourself the facts about teen sexuality in your community.
- *Help your teen understand the internal and external pressures to express their sexuality and to make responsible decisions*—In other words, your teen needs to know where you stand. You need to share your hopes for your teen's future as well as your concerns for the day-to-day issues your teen may be facing.
- *Make sure that your teen knows the facts about pregnancy and sexually transmitted diseases (STDs) like HIV-AIDS*—No teen should be without this basic health information. If you can't provide the information yourself—for whatever reason—find someone who can, and ask them to talk with your teen.
- *Be there for your teen, no matter what*—Teens tend to live for today. Discussions you and your teen have, and decisions you make together, will be tested by time and events in your teen's life. Don't fool yourself about the fears and pressures your teen may face on a daily basis. Sometimes teens

are more capable intellectually than they are emotionally. Let your teen know that you will always be there, no matter what happens.

Guidelines

Educating your teen about sex is a process—that much should be clear already. It should also be clear that waiting to talk about sex until you think your teen is involved in a relationship—or even waiting until he or she starts dating—is not a good idea. Look at it this way: your teen is going to hear a lot more of what you have to say when he or she isn't distracted. As with many things, timing is everything when it comes to talking about sex. Don't panic, but don't wait, is a good rule of thumb. The guidelines below can help, too.

- *Don't say everything at once*—Remember, your goal is to help your teen develop healthy attitudes and behaviors, and that takes time. A single barrage of information—or worse yet a check list of do's and don'ts—is just an updated version of the old "The Birds and the Bees" lecture. Sure, you may need some sort of ice-breaker discussion, but be sure to let your teen know that talking to you about sex is not a one-time thing.
- *Respect your teen's privacy and respect your own privacy*—Intimate details don't have to be part of a useful discussion about sex. You can respect your teen's privacy by keeping your discussion rather general and objective to start. If your teen confides in you, keep what is said in

confidence. Try to remember what it was like when you were a teen. And remember, conversations about sex with your teen aren't about you or the details of your sex life. In fact, most teens don't want to know about their parent's sex life. What teens want is information and education about what is happening in *their* lives.

- *Talk about options, consequences, and planning*—Educating your teen about sex is not a one-way street. As with any learning, both teacher and student must be involved. Keep your teen involved by working through the facts and issues, not by judging or claiming to always know best.

Taking an Active Role

Too many parents behave as though teenagers are adults and are ready to make adult decisions. Just because your teenagers express a need for independence, does not mean that they have automatically acquired the maturity to handle that independence. The following rules may seem obvious, but it is distressing to see how many parents are afraid to enforce them. Teens are much more likely to thrive in a structured environment than in a situation where they are not sure of the rules and are unclear about what behavior is appropriate, and what behavior is not.

- Know where your teen is and who your teen is with.
- Know your teen's friends.
- If your teen is visiting a friend, make sure that a responsible adult is present.
- Set a reasonable curfew.

Head Off Trouble

Teen pregnancy can ravage a young person's life. So can HIV/AIDS. Some of the early indicators of trouble include the following.

Early dating: The likelihood of teen pregnancy and of sexually transmitted diseases is much greater for teens who start to date before the age of fourteen or fifteen. *Frequent* dating in the later teen years is also a trouble indicator.

Trouble in school: Teens who are frequently in trouble with their teachers and school officials are also at greater risk than those who are not in trouble.

Use of alcohol and tobacco: Use of alcohol and tobacco is much more frequent than use of illegal drugs among teens. Use of any of these substances is highly related to teen pregnancy and sexually transmitted diseases, probably because such use indicates problem peers.

Very poor grades in school: Frustrating school performance should obviously be dealt with for its own sake. In addition, school failure often leads teens to seek alternative sources of gratification, and those alternatives are potential bombs when they involve sexual activity.

Although the early indicators listed above can help parents and other caring adults spot problems, teen pregnancy and sexually transmitted disease can also affect teens who do well, are active in school, and who do not use alcohol and tobacco. Do not assume that your son or daughter doesn't need your guidance. Encourage open discussions about sex, and make your values, opinions, experience, and advice known. You can only influence your teen's behavior if you are actively involved.

Helping your teen to develop a strong sense of self, high self-esteem, and a compelling belief in respectable values and ethical behavior, and encouraging him or her to set personal goals for the future are the best things you can do to prevent irresponsible sexual behavior.

The Case for Abstinence

Health officials describe *abstinence* as "choosing not to engage in certain behaviors such as sexual intercourse or drug use." While every teen should know the guidelines for safe sexual contact and the dangers of drugs and alcohol—if for no other reason than as a public health and safety issue—abstinence is a different matter. Abstinence means making a commitment and consistently avoiding certain behaviors—any time, any day, and under any circumstances.

To date, there is no known cure for HIV/AIDS. For many people, that fact alone is enough to make a case for abstinence to their teen. For other people, the facts about HIV/AIDS are only part of larger picture that makes abstinence for their teen the right idea.

Obviously, your stance on abstinence is a personal one. No one wants to put their child at risk to life-threatening situations. Most people, however, still struggle with finding appropriate behaviors that allow

teens to express intimacy, caring, and love. It is this gray area that adults and teens need to thoroughly explore together: On the one hand saying absolutely "no" to certain behaviors while, on the other hand, having normal feelings of caring and sharing. Your teen wants to hear from you how to grow and develop into an adult. Abstinence is an adult issue, and like many adult issues, it takes strength, caring, compassion, and discipline, often in equal measures and at nearly the same time. Working with your teen on abstinence and other adult issues on a regular basis is a powerful a gift to give to your teen.

Sexually Transmitted Diseases

It may be hard to accept, but your child's sexual activity can be too dangerous to ignore. Sexually transmitted diseases (STDs) are at an all time high. Every year, three million teenagers are infected with an STD.

An STD is a bacterial or viral infection that is passed from one person to another through sexual contact. Two-thirds of STD cases are in the under-25 age group. There are more than twenty-five highly contagious STDs. Genital sores and irritations from STDs are an opening for the HIV virus that causes AIDS. Some STDs can be cured or controlled with medications. Untreated, some STDs can lead to sterility, brain damage, cancer, or death. Many STDs have few or no symptoms.

Young people aged fifteen to nineteen have a higher rate of gonorrhea than other age groups according to the Centers for Disease Control and Prevention. The rate of other sexually-transmitted diseases, such as chlamydia and herpes, is growing as well. Twenty to 30 percent of sexually active teenaged women may have chlamydia. Those at greatest risk live in urban areas. Women are more likely than men to get STDs and yet are less likely to seek care.

Young people get the message everywhere—from movies and music to billboards and beer commercials—that sex will make them popular, smarter, and more attractive. Yet the real risks are rarely presented. That's where parents and guardians come in. Although sexuality is a normal, healthy part of life, young teens need to understand that the decision to have intercourse can affect the rest of their lives. Intercourse increases the risk of becoming pregnant or getting a potentially fatal disease. Young teens also need to hear that sex has emotional risks, like feeling guilty or regretful because having sex is against the morals and values of their families.

Teens have a hard time asking direct questions about sex. Don't wait. Bring up the topic. Use plots from TV, movies, public service announcements, and lyrics from songs as springboards. Teens often ask indirect questions and use a friend's problems to get at their concerns. Listen carefully. Studies show that teens look to parents or caregivers as their most important source of information about sex, but that parents often let them down. Your teen does care about what you think, feel, and value. Teens say the major reason they don't wait until they

---

The Most Common STD's

Chlamydia—Similar to gonorrhea, but has symptoms in men and is asymptomatic in women.

Genital Warts—Highly contagious. Caused by the human papilloma virus (HPV). Symptoms include genital irritation, itching, and warts. Has been linked to cervical cancer.

Gonorrhea—Teens have more cases than other age groups. Symptoms include genital discharge and discomfort while urinating. New drug-resistant strains have made penicillin ineffective. Can cause pelvic inflammatory disease and sterility.

Herpes—Causes clusters of painful blisters. No cure, but there is advancement in treating and controlling symptoms. Can cause serious illness or death to a newborn during delivery.

Syphilis—Increasing among teens. Starts with sore or chancre on the genitals. The sore will disappear but the disease will not. Untreated, it can cause brain damage, heart disease, and eventually death. Can be treated with penicillin.

---

are older to have sex is they feel pressured by other teens.

The Centers for Disease Control and Prevention reported in a 1992 study that 45 percent of fifteen-year-olds were sexually active. But teens need to hear that *not everybody* is having sex. Today, there are signs that abstinence is gaining favor with young teens. More teens are dating in groups, rather than in pairs. This way, kids can make friends with the opposite sex without pressure to become intimate.

Families can help teens avoid making a casual decision about sex by talking about the importance of meaningful relationships. When kids understand family values, they are more able to deal with pressure by peers. In the long run, teenagers adopt their parents' attitudes. If you never tell them what you think, how will they know? A good long-term goal is to teach your kids how to make decisions and to deal with pressure when you're not there.

Teens and HIV/AIDS

AIDS is the sixth leading cause of death among people ages 15 through 24. The fastest growing segment of the population infected with HIV—the virus that causes AIDS—are young adults ages 13 through 24. Those two facts alone highlight the importance of HIV/AIDS education. Consider a few other important facts.

- Since there is no cure for HIV/AIDS, prevention is the only way to stop the spread of the disease.
- Since AIDS can take years to develop after someone is infected with the HIV virus, a diagnosis of AIDS as a young adult means that the disease was probably transmitted during adolescence.

- Substance abuse can increase a teen's risk for contracting AIDS because many teens take chances with unsafe sex when their judgment is impaired by drugs or alcohol.

Michigan legislation mandates HIV/AIDS education for public school students in grades kindergarten through twelve. Topics that may be taught to teens in grades nine and ten are how HIV/AIDS is similar and different from other communicable diseases, levels of infection, and prevention from contracting HIV by abstinent behavior. In grades eleven and twelve, topics may include: Identifying and reducing high risk situations, facts and myths about AIDS and AIDS testing, as well as ethical, political, and economic issues.

Basic Facts about HIV/AIDS

Before you talk with your teen, it is important for you to have the basic facts about the disease. AIDS stands for Acquired Immune Deficiency Syndrome. In other words, AIDS is not hereditary, but Acquired from the environment. AIDS attacks the Immune system, creating a Deficiency in how the body fights infections and disease. The group of symptoms indicating the presence of the disease is known as a Syndrome.

AIDS is spread through *blood contact* with a person infected with the HIV virus. Three body fluids that are known to transmit HIV are blood, semen, and vaginal fluid. People usually contract AIDS in the following ways.

- By having sex with someone infected with HIV.
- By sharing drug equipment, especially needles, used by a person with the HIV virus.
- By sharing devices used for tattooing or ear piercing with someone infected with HIV.
- AIDS can also be contracted by blood contaminated with the HIV virus and used in blood transfusions, although this is becoming more and more rare.
- A pregnant woman infected with HIV can pass the virus to her baby during pregnancy or delivery.

There are many myths about HIV/AIDS. Here are some facts: HIV is a relatively weak virus. The virus can only live in a few kinds of cells and dies very quickly when outside the body. The virus *cannot* be transmitted by casual contact, by hugging, or through mosquito bites. The virus *cannot* be transmitted by sharing telephones, a toilet seat, a drinking fountain, a swimming pool, or by social kissing.

AIDS can only detected through a blood test that checks for HIV infection. Your doctor or county health department can provide information on where to obtain HIV testing. To date there is no vaccine against AIDS and no known cure for the disease.

Talking with Your Teen

Talking to your teen about HIV/AIDS can be difficult and uncomfortable. The disease is linked to sexual behavior and drug use— subjects that touch the core of most adults' personal and cultural values.

In any discussion about HIV/AIDS, you need to emphasize the potential threat of the disease to the life of your teen, as well as the need for education and prevention. Adults need to know that talking about sex— whether abstinence or the correct way to use a condom—does not encourage promiscuity in teens. In fact, several studies have shown that sexual activity among teens decreased or remained the same after being involved in sex education programs that included information about condoms. Your teen needs to hear three important messages about HIV/AIDS directly from you.

- Many teens practice sexual behaviors that increase their risk for contracting HIV and other sexually transmitted diseases (STDs).
- Every year, 3 million American teens contract an STD. One in four sexually active teens will contract an STD by the time he or she reaches 21. Some STDs may increase the risk of contracting HIV by creating skin lesions that make it easier to acquire the virus.
- By age twenty, 86 percent of men and 77 percent of women have had sexual intercourse, and 19 percent of all high school students have had four or more partners. The median age of reported first intercourse is 16.9 years for females and 16.1 years for males.

Studies by the FDA Center for Devices and Radiological Health confirm that latex condoms are a highly effective barrier to HIV-sized particles. *Latex condoms* are the only contraceptive labeled by the FDA to be effective in preventing sexual transmission of HIV.

Here are a few suggestions for starting a discussion about HIV/AIDS.

- Ask your teen what he or she is learning about HIV/AIDS in health class, or other classes. Your teen's answer can be the starting point of a conversation.
- Look to newspapers, magazines, radio, movies, and television for stories and advertisements about HIV/AIDS that you can use as a discussion starter.
- Local events such as health fairs or AIDS benefits are often a good place families and teens to learn about the disease. Use such events as educational experiences for both you and your teen.

Talking with your teen about HIV/AIDS is too important to give up on if your first attempt is cut short. Don't worry about saying everything at once, and don't worry about changing how you bring up the subject. Have patience and understand that talking about HIV/AIDS is a process. After all, you're talking about helping your teen make a lifetime of informed decisions.

The AIDS Epidemic Today

Scientific data suggests that at least 40,000 Americans are being infected with HIV each year. About the same number of people die each year from HIV related illnesses. So, roughly speaking, for every person who dies from HIV related illnesses, another person becomes infected with HIV. Researchers estimate that the number of people living with HIV has remained about the same since 1990. Given these

statistics, each new generation of teens faces the same need for HIV/AIDS education. Worldwide, the AIDS epidemic continues to grow. Again, the message to teens needs to be for education and prevention of HIV/AIDS.

The Fourth Conference on Retroviruses and Opportunitstic Infections held in late January, 1997, in Washington, DC, ended with hope that some of the experimental drugs for HIV/AIDS reported on at the conference will ultimately ease the burden of patients who must stick with a difficult schedule when taking the drugs currently available.

Writing in the *New York Times* (January 27, 1997; page A-8), Lawrence K. Altman described the conference.

> Speakers at the meeting, which drew more than 2,300 AIDS experts and other scientists, said they had been astonished by the favorable turn of events since last year's AIDS conference, when combination drug therapies were first shown to be able to suppress HIV, the virus that causes AIDS, below the limits of detection. The combination therapies use older drugs like AZT and a new class of drugs, protease inhibitors.
>
> The wider use of various combinations, including some that do not include protease inhibitors, are now promising to transform AIDS into a chronic disease that is manageable.
>
> Nevertheless, speaker after speaker said that drugs would not end the worldwide AIDS epidemic, in part because poor countries could not afford their cost. The only hope for denting the

global epidemic is a vaccine against HIV, but no breakthroughs in HIV vaccine research were reported at the meeting.

From the same conference, Shankar Vedantam, *Detroit Free Press* Washington Staff, reported the following in the January 23, 1997, edition (page 5A).

"Can HIV be eradicated from an infected person?" David Ho, one of the country's most celebrated AIDS researchers, asked Wednesday at the opening of the five-day conference. "The answer is, we don't know."

In hundreds of patients, HIV has been driven down to levels so low that scientists can find no trace of it in patients' blood. Still, researchers know that the virus is hiding in some organs and tissues and fear that if they halt treatment, it will return. . . .

"In general," said Douglas Richman, chairman of the conference's scientific program committee and an AIDS researcher, "patients who showed suppression (of the virus) at one to two years, and who are still taking their medicines, are still suppressed at two to three years.". . .

Some 8,500 people are infected with the virus every day, said Peter Piot, chief of the United Nations Joint Program on AIDS. Thirty million are now infected worldwide, and last year, 1.5 million people died of AIDS.

HIV/AIDS Statistics

Figures from June, 1996, indicate that 548,102 cases of AIDS had been reported in the United States. Of those cases, approximately 343,000 have died.

Figures indicate that between 650,000 and 900,000 Americans are infected with HIV.

According to a study from the Centers for Disease Control and Prevention, 42,506 Americans died of AIDS in 1995. (As of January 31, 1997, there are no nationwide statistics available for 1996.)

For information about support groups for HIV positive patients, contact *AIDS Partnership Michigan Client Services* at 1-800-515-3434.

Contributions and review by Eli Saltz, Ph.D., Director, The Merrill-Palmer Institute, Detroit, Michigan.

Reviewed by:

Patricia Nichols, M.S., C.H.E.S., Supervisor of Comprehensive Programs in Health & Early Childhood, Michigan Department of Education, Lansing, Michigan.

Randall S. Pope, Chief, HIV/AIDS Prevention & Intervention, Michigan Department of Community Health, Lansing, Michigan.

Joy Schumacher, RN, BSN, Oakland County Health Department AIDS Office, Pontiac, Michigan.

Donald B. Sweeney, M.A., Chief, School Health Unit, Michigan Department of Community Health, Lansing, Michigan.

Chapter 11

TEENS AND SEXUAL HARASSMENT

What is Harassment?

Your teen may face unwanted sexual attention from another student, a teacher, a coach, or a boss. We used to just ignore this type of behavior, but now we know that sexual harassment is unfair and should not be tolerated. You can help by educating your son or daughter to understand what sexual harassment is. Your teen should also know that she or he should report unwanted sexual attention to you or another trusted adult rather than keeping it a secret. Both girls and boys should be aware of sexual harassment and how to prevent it.

One reason parents give for not talking about sexual harassment with their teens is that they don't understand it. Sexual harassment is unwanted sexual attention at school or at work, and usually takes one or more of the following forms.

- *Physical*: Unwanted pinching, brushing against the body, kissing, touching, or rape.
- *Verbal*: Sexual or derogatory jokes, comments, or conversations.
- *Pictorial*: Sexual pictures, graffiti, or cartoons.
- *Sensory*: Leering, gestures, or whistling.

Although girls are more frequently sexually harassed, teenage boys are vulnerable, too. Here are some examples.

- Another teen in your daughter's class makes frequent comments about her breast size and asks her whether she's "done it."
- Another student posts a sexual cartoon on your teen's locker.
- Your son's coach suggestively rubs up against him during practice and asks him to stay late to train alone with him.
- Your daughter's teacher tells her that he will give her an "A" if she will make out with him.

Effects of Harassment

Sexual harassment in schools is a widespread problem. One recent study of students in grades eight to eleven found that 85 percent of girls have experienced sexual harassment, and of those girls, 65 percent were touched, grabbed, or pinched in a sexual way. Another study of teen girls found that 83 percent were touched, pinched, or grabbed, and that 39 percent were sexually harassed at school on a daily basis in the last year. Peer harassment (one student harassing another student) is the most common form of sexual harassment in the schools.

Sexual harassment can have devastating effects on teens. It can cause serious educational, emotional, and physical problems for students and create a barrier to full and equal participation in education. Studies show that 33 percent of girls who were sexually harassed say they do not want to attend school; 32 percent report not wanting to talk as much in class; 28 percent found it harder to pay attention in school; and 18 percent report that it made them think about changing schools. In addition, 64 percent of girls who have been harassed report being embarrassed; 52 percent report feeling self-conscious; 43 percent felt less sure or less confident about themselves; and 30 percent doubted whether they could ever have a happy romantic relationship. Teens suffer even more if their school fails to deal with the problem of sexual harassment.

Some of the most common responses of teens who experience sexual harassment are to deny it to themselves, blame themselves, begin to avoid people and situations, and decide to do nothing. If they decide to do nothing, the harassment often increases. Getting your teen to tell you about being harassed is the first step toward solving the problem.

Support Your Teen

Be open with your teen so that he or she comes to you about sexual harassment. Do not judge how your teen dealt with the harassment. Listen carefully and let your teen know that you are on his or her side. Express your support and that you are proud that he or she told you about the harassment.

Get help for your teen and make sure that the harassment stops. Call your teen's school or place of work where the harassment happened. Meet with the principal or company manager to discuss the problem. Request that disciplinary action be taken against the harasser if that is appropriate. Seek professional help for your teen from a source you trust. A counselor or other mental health

professional can help you decide what type of help, if any, your teen may need. In severe cases, you may want to contact an attorney to discuss your teen's legal rights.

Your Role

One of your most important roles as a parent is to teach your children to respect others and to treat them equally and fairly. You serve as a role model for your teen. Your own values, attitudes, and behavior tell your teen how to treat others. To stop sexual harassment before it happens, teach your children respect for women, men, girls, and boys. Show them that it is not right to tell sexual jokes at school or at work. Teach them that no one can touch their bodies without their permission. Help your teen learn the facts about sexual harassment through your actions as well as your words.

Education and Prevention

Prompt and effective attention to the problem of sexual harassment can reduce both its frequency and its devastating effects. Most schools have a policy regarding sexual harassment. Work with your child's school to ensure that students are protected. A model policy would include the following.

- A clear definition and statement of policy against sexual harassment.
- Programs to educate students and teachers about sexual harassment and the school's policy.
- Information about how to file a complaint.

- A procedure so that complaints are handled in a fair and timely manner.
- A guarantee of confidentiality to the extent possible under the circumstances.
- A promise by the school to act quickly to end sexual harassment and to impose appropriate discipline where necessary.

By working with your child's school, you can help prevent sexual harassment and send a message to students and the community that it is not acceptable behavior.

Written by Holly Fechner, J.D., Labor and Employment Attorney, Policy Office of the U.S. Department of Labor, Washington, DC.

Reviewed by Helene Mills, Ed.D., Principal, Seaholm High School, Birmingham, Michigan.

Chapter 12

TEEN SAFETY AND CRIME PREVENTION

Awareness First

Teens are of the age when they can be away from their families and be more independent—going places with friends or going alone. This new-found freedom becomes a problem for some teens because they feel invulnerable—they take risks. The key to increasing your teen's safety away from home is *awareness*. The more aware your teen is of possible dangers, the safer he or she will be.

In the teenage years, the desire to belong or fit in is especially strong, which may make your son or daughter go along with unsafe activities, or reluctant to leave an unsafe situation. Share the following information with your teen and help him or her understand that being aware is smart, and will help them stay safe.

Statistics show that people who think about possible crime situations and plan what they would do ahead of time are better off. First, they are more aware of their surroundings and therefore are much less likely to be chosen as targets. Second, they are more likely to be able to keep their wits about them and escape without serious injury if they are attacked.

Sexual Assault

Sexual assault is any sexual act committed by one person against another without that person's consent. No matter what it is called—sexual assault, sexual abuse, or date, acquaintance, or stranger rape—such conduct is against the law and is *never* the survivor's fault.

Michigan law recognizes four degrees of sexual assault, depending on whether the assault consisted of penetration or of contact without penetration, and on the relationship between the assailant and the victim. The legal term for sexual assault in Michigan is *criminal sexual conduct*, which puts this crime in its proper perspective and creates a clear-cut distinction between the criminal and the victim.

Sexual assault is a crime of violence and degradation, and has nothing to do with lust or sex or love, and is *never* the survivor's fault. Force is a part of any sexual assault, which can be in the form of emotional coercion, implicit threats, verbal threats, or physical force with or without a weapon. Rape is always the responsibility of the rapist, *not* the person being attacked.

Rape Awareness and Prevention

Few people would say to a victim of armed robbery, "You had it coming." Unfortunately, our society has long blamed sexual assault on the victim. The facts about sexual assault show an entirely different picture.

- One in four women is sexually assaulted before the age of eighteen.
- One in three women, and one in eight men will be sexually assaulted at some time in his or her lifetime.

- Most sexual offenders are someone the targeted person knows and trusts.
- Survivors of sexual assault do not lie about the crime. False reports of sexual assault occur at the same rate as any other crime.

Dating and Sexual Assault

Rape is an unpleasant subject—even more so in dating relationships. We don't want to think about it. We don't want to talk about it. We don't want to believe that this violent crime could happen to us or someone we love. Please review the information below very carefully, and then discuss it thoroughly with your teen. Help him or her develop an understanding of the facts about date or "acquaintance" rape. Many such crimes go unreported because the survivors feel they somehow invited the attack by going out with the perpetrator. Although this crime is most often committed against women and girls, teenage boys are vulnerable, too (to attack by men or other boys). Most people find it unbelievable, but boys are at great risk because *they do not even consider it a possibility,* and *have no idea what to do.* The element of surprise works in the criminal's favor. Young men are also the least likely to report a rape because of the shame involved.

Your teenager needs to know that sexual assault *can* happen in relationships. Talk with your teen about sexual assault before they start going out with other teens in groups or on dates. Tell your teen that, no matter what the circumstances were that led up to the assault, rape is never his or her fault. Not all

rapes can be prevented, but taking some precautions can reduce the risk. Teach your son or daughter these rules.

- Know what your sexual limits and values are. Make sure you have it clear in your mind whether, with whom, and under what circumstances you would engage in sexual behavior, and how much.
- *No always means NO.* It doesn't matter what the circumstances are, who the person is, or how you feel at the time; no means no. It is never OK to force yourself on someone. If someone tries to force themselves on you, it is OK to defend yourself.
- *Speak up immediately!* Silence can be misinterpreted as consent. Communicate to your date your intent and expectations about dating and sexual limits. State your feelings clearly and firmly.
- *Stay alert.* Drug and alcohol use, besides being illegal, reduce a person's ability to evaluate potentially dangerous situations.
- *Act on your gut feelings.* Leave an uncomfortable situation—you do not owe anyone anything.
- *Do what it takes to stay safe.* Scream, yell, or get angry if you must. If people are nearby, yell, "FIRE!" to get their attention (you may want to practice yelling and screaming).

Self-defense Strategies

There is no single plan or tactic that will work in every assault situation. Your teen needs to know that his or her gut feelings about a situation may be the most important self-defense tool he or she has. Your son, especially, needs to understand that it is possible for him to be sexually assaulted, and that awareness is a means of protecting himself. Discuss these points with your teen.

- *Trust your instincts.* If a situation feels unsafe, it probably is. Stay calm and do not panic—concentrate on your breathing to keep from freezing up. *Take your inner feelings seriously and react quickly.*
- *Get away.* If at all possible, get away to somewhere safe and seek help immediately. Never stay in a situation that makes you uncomfortable, whether that is on a date or while walking home alone. Always carry enough money for a phone call and a bus or cab fare home.
- *Talk to the attacker.* Most rapists report that they never considered the victim a *person.* Talk about family and parents, or tell the rapist he is hurting you. You may make him see you as more than an object. (Some people have escaped sexual assault by telling the attacker that they have HIV/AIDS or another sexually transmitted disease.)
- *Make a scene if other people are nearby.* It is perfectly acceptable to shout out loud, "THIS MAN IS BOTHERING ME!" or "GET YOUR DAMN HANDS OFF ME!"
- *As a last resort: Fight back.* Fighting back *may* stop the assault and create a moment for the you to get away, or fighting may increase the intensity of the attack. There is no set rule because every situation is different: Use your best judgment. Statistics do show that survivors who fought back were

more likely to *stop* the attack. If you decide to fight back, no tactic should be attempted half-way—you must use all the strength you have to create a chance to get away.

Don't Give Up

There is no one "right" solution or guarantee in a sexual assault, but survivors who *don't give up* have a much greater chance of escaping. Not all people are physically or emotionally prepared to defend themselves in an assault. Generally, unless people (this includes adult males) have had a chance to think through and/or practice self-defense tactics, they will be at a disadvantage in a hand-to-hand fight with a criminal.

Self-defense classes may help your teen feel more confident about using a physical response. Ideally, families should advocate for personal protection classes as part of a school's physical education curriculum. Rape crisis programs and community education programs may also have information on self-defense resources.

Detroit News columnist, J.B. Dixon reports the results of a Channel 7 (Detroit) survey of rapists revealed that 60 percent would stop an attack if the victim fought back; 63 percent would be stopped by a liquid tear gas or pepper spray, and 67 percent would be stopped by a whistle or alarm.

If Your Teen is Assaulted

Sexual assault is a traumatic and sometimes life-threatening crime. If your teen tells you that she or he has been sexually assaulted, believe him or her, and don't blame your teen for the attack. Teens are often victimized while doing something they aren't supposed to be doing, such as sneaking out of the house, going to a party when they said they were babysitting, or going out with someone they just met at the mall. It is the lie and fear of getting in trouble that may keep a teen from disclosing a rape (both males and females). Even if this is the case, your teen is not responsible for the attack—the *rapist* is responsible.

Don't let shock, anger, or embarrassment keep you from getting your teen immediate help. You may wish to first call a 24-hour rape crisis hotline for advice on getting help. (Check your Yellow Pages under Crisis Intervention, Hotlines & Helping Lines (after Hotels) or call your hospital or telephone information for a local center.) Most crisis centers have victim assistance programs that will help you get medical assistance, contact the police, and get other professional support. The steps below are recommended in any case of sexual assault.

* *Report the assault to the police in the city in which the crime occurred.*

This step should be taken *with your teen's consent* as soon as possible after the attack. Talking with the police may be painful for your teen, and you. Keep in mind, however, that your teen has done nothing wrong and may not be the attacker's only victim.

If your son or daughter is reluctant to report the crime to police, a rape crisis

counselor can help address any questions or fears you or your teen may have about reporting, and may even be able to accompany you to the police station.

* *Seek medical attention at a hospital or medical center as soon as possible after the assault.*

Medical attention is important for several reasons. First, the exam will help determine if your teen has been physically injured in any way. Second, physical evidence will be collected, which will be preserved for possible prosecution. Avoid letting your teen bathe or shower until after the exam, and bring the clothes that were worn during the assault to the hospital.

The hospital exam will include testing for sexually transmitted diseases. For privacy purposes, you may choose to have HIV/AIDS testing conducted at some other site, such as your County Health Department. If your son or daughter is in an intimate relationship, be sure that you or medical staff discuss the need to practice safe sex pending the outcome of the test results.

The exam will include a pregnancy test if the victim is a woman. If you or your teen have concerns about unwanted pregnancy, discuss this issue with the examiners and ask about the morning after pill.

Most insurance policies will cover the medical exam. If you are uninsured, you may be eligible for crime victim compensation. Your local rape crisis program or Prosecuting Attorney's office can help you file a claim.

Recovering from an Assault

Your teen needs your love and support after surviving a sexual assault. Fear, depression, anxiety, embarrassment, and feeling powerless are not uncommon among survivors. Your teen may have problems thinking or concentrating. School or work performance may suffer. She or he may become physically ill, be afraid to leave the house, or not want to be touched by anyone. Some teens need professional guidance to work out feelings of anger, shame, and guilt. A counselor from a rape crisis program or a mental health professional can help you decide what kind of help your teen may need.

Family members also suffer after an assault. You may blame yourself for not having protected your teen. You may want to restrict your teen's freedom in the hope that it will prevent further victimization. You may find your teen's behavior toward you is confusing and hurtful. You may fear your teen is "damaged" for life. You need support, too. Talking to a rape crisis counselor or a trusted friend can help you sort out your feelings so that you are better prepared to help your son or daughter recover from sexual assault.

Sexual Abuse

Between 70 and 80 percent of the sexual abuse of young people is by someone they know, trust, or even love. To make matters worse, very few survivors feel able to tell anyone about the abuse. Fear, shame, and confusion often combine to allow the sexual abuse to continue for months and even years. In addition, the attention that the child receives may be filling a void and, therefore, feel satisfying to the child since sexual abuse is usually seductive and not brutish.

Parents, families members, and caring adults need to know—and admit to themselves—that sexual abuse can happen to the child or teen they love. The unthinkable can happen. When children are still young, it is important to teach them the concepts of "good" touches and "bad" touches, and to give them a sense that they have a personal space that is not to be violated by anyone. A strong sense of self-worth and personal value enables a child or teen to rebuke this type of overture. In fact, such an overture will probably not be made to a confident child.

Children and teens need to know that they can come to their parents or a caring adult about any situation that makes them feel uncomfortable. Finally, *you* need to understand that sexual abuse is never your child's or teen's fault. You must be prepared to hear that an uncle, a sibling, a teacher, or your spouse is abusing your child and not blame your child.

Signs of Abuse

Physical signs of sexual abuse may include having sexually transmitted diseases such as gonorrhea or syphilis at a young age. Torn skin in and around the vagina, swelling of the genitals, foul vaginal or anal odor, frequent urination or a painful or burning sensation during urination may also be signs of sexual abuse. Sometimes, pregnancy at age twelve or younger is a sign.

Behavioral signs may include acting in sexually seductive ways or talking about sexual things in a more mature manner than appropriate for their age. Some teens may have poor relationships with peers or start fighting at school, or fail to finish school assignments and get low grades.

A teen may also exhibit the following.

- Act pseudo-mature.
- Become depressed.
- Become angry.
- Use drugs and/or alcohol.
- Become self-destructive.
- Have a marked decrease in self-esteem.

The reaction to sexual abuse varies with the individual. It should be noted that some survivors of sexual abuse may react by focusing all of their energy into school work and making the honor roll—becoming the "model" child.

Most victims, however, act out in negative ways. They may run away, have sex with many different individuals (become promiscuous), either think about or attempt suicide, or turn to alcohol and other drug use. A teen may have no friends visit the home, and have problems trusting others. If abused at home, they may spend more time away from home or avoid being around the abuser elsewhere.

A female may become ashamed of her body or develop an eating disorder such as anorexia or bulimia. Girls who have been abused have also been known to mutilate themselves by repeatedly scratching their bodies or biting their lips, nails, fingers, or mouth until they bleed.

Males and females may begin to lie, steal, and get into fights. Despite the lack of correlation, boys may fear becoming homosexual if abused by a male. Boys most often do not tell anyone that they have been abused. Boys also believe they cannot possibly be victims—they must always be brave—and exhibit a macho behavior.

If Your Teen Has Been Abused

Children and teens seldom lie about sexual abuse. Your role is to listen carefully and let your teen know that you are very angry at the abuser and not at your child. Let your teen know that you love him or her. It is important not to ask your teen what role they may have played in the abuse. Don't blame the innocent. Above all, your son or daughter needs to know that you are on his or her side, no matter what.

Getting assistance for your teen and your family is the important next step. Call the police. If your son or daughter has been abused, there are likely to be other victims. Seek professional help from a source you trust. Your doctor, religious institution, or school may be able to provide a referral. Check with your local family service agency, crisis center, or community mental health services agency. Children's Protective Services—listed in the phone book, can also help.

"Sexual Assault" *modified with permission from the* Citizens Against Crime *program on personal crime prevention (Allen, Texas: 1-800-466-1010).*

Contributions to and review of "Sexual Assault" by Gloria Krys, M.A., C.S.W., L.P.C., Program Coordinator of the Assault Crisis Center of Washtenaw County Community Mental Health (1866 Packard Road, Ypsilanti, Michigan 48197. 24-hour Crisis line: 313-483-7273).

"Sexual Assault" *reviewed by:*

Jerry Aris, President of Citizens Against Crime, Allen, Texas.

Patsy Baker, Program Analyst, Rape Prevention and Services Program, Child & Family Services, Michigan Family Independence Agency, Lansing, Michigan.

Laurie Bechhofer, MPH Evaluation Consultant, Supervisor, Comprehensive Programs in Health & Childhood, Michigan Department of Education, Lansing, Michigan.

Sue Coats, Program Director of Turning Point, Mt. Clemens, Michigan.

Althea Grant, Executive Director of the Detroit Rape Crisis Center, Detroit Receiving Hospital, Detroit, Michigan.

Ellen Hayse, Resource Coordinator for the Resource Center on Sexual and Domestic Violence, Lansing, Michigan.

Auleen A. Jarrett, President of CRIMEFREE Seminars, Inc., Livonia, Michigan.

Rachel N. Kay, M.P.H., Cook County Department of Public Health, Oak Park, Illinois.

Helene Mills, Ed.D., Principal, Seaholm High School, Birmingham, Michigan.

Sherry Murphy, Oakland Schools Intermediate School District, Waterford, Michigan.

Donald B. Sweeney, Chief, School Health Unit, Michigan Department of Community Health, Lansing, Michigan.

"Sexual Abuse" *modified from* Teen to Teen: Personal Safety and Sexual Abuse Prevention *by Catalina Herrerias, MSW, Ph.D. (KIDSRIGHTS, 10100 Park Cedar Drive, Charlotte, NC 28210; 1-800-892-5437, 1993). Reprinted with permission of the publisher.*

"Sexual Abuse" *reviewed by:*

Gloria Krys, MA, C.S.W., L.P.C., Program Coordinator, Assault Crisis Center of Washtenaw County Community Mental Health (1866 Packard Road, Ypsilanti, Michigan 48197. 24-hour Crisis line: 313-483-7273).

Betty Tableman, M.P.A., Director, Prevention Services, Michigan Department of Community Health, Lansing, Michigan.

Second edition contributions and review by Naomi Haines Griffith, M.A., M.S.W., Executive Director, Parents and Children Together (PACT), Consultant, Alabama Children's Trust Fund, Decatur, Alabama.

Chapter 13

TEENS AND VIOLENCE

The Face of Violence

In recent years, violence seems to define the United States. Forget the daily headlines, the celebrity trials, and even—for a moment—your own experience, to consider a single fact: The United States has one of the highest civilian homicide rates of any country in the world. When compared to twenty-one other developed nations, not only are U.S. homicides staggering in terms of lost human life—some 25,000 Americans are killed each year—the homicide rate for 15-24 year old males in the U.S. is nearly *four* times greater than the next nation surveyed.

Children and adolescents are especially affected by violence. Over 2,000 children and adolescents die violent deaths each year. Another 1.5 million children suffer abuse and neglect. To make matters worse, the character of violence involving children and adolescents has changed in recent years.

- Homicide is the most common cause of death in young African American males *and* females.
- Handguns are widely available to adolescents. In 75 percent of all teen homicides, a handgun is involved.
- Children and teens are becoming violent and committing violent crimes at an earlier and earlier age. Huge numbers of first and second graders say they have witnessed violent crimes. The juvenile courts are crowded with murder cases involving 10-year-olds and young adolescents.

Violence at Home

Underlying all of the statistics and tragedy of violence in the United States is a single, long-standing truth: *the single greatest predictor of future violence is a previous history of violence.* In other words, violence begins where children first learn: in the home. This single truth makes domestic violence a matter of public health at the very least, and a matter of national concern if Americans want to break the cycle of violence.

What Is Domestic Violence?

To most people, domestic violence is a husband hitting a wife, or a drunken boyfriend slapping around his girlfriend in the middle of the night. Such simple stereotypes distort what is really behind domestic violence—one partner's need for power and control in the relationship. The force used can be physical, sexual, or emotional/psychological.

Domestic violence is a pattern of learned behavior in which one person uses force to control another person. Such behavior often consists of frequent—even daily—instances of abuse. Criminal behaviors including assault, sexual abuse, and stalking, are against the law. Emotional, psychological, and financial abuse, although generally not begun as criminal behaviors, may lead to, or be part of criminal behaviors.

Michigan law defines domestic violence as "an assault upon the victim who is the abuser's spouse, former spouse, or a person residing or having resided in the same household, or a person having a child in common with the abuser." Below are a few examples of the many forms domestic violence can take, including forms not covered by the laws.

- Hitting, slapping, biting, or burning one's partner.
- Causing injuries such as bruises, black eyes, broken bones, or broken teeth.
- Holding, tying down, or restraining one's partner against his or her will.
- Using a weapon to threaten to injure one's partner.
- Threatening to injure or kill one's partner or the partner's children, family members, friends, or pets.
- Forcing one's partner to have sex or engage in unwanted sexual activities.
- Destroying household or personal belongings and/or hurting or killing pets.
- Preventing one's partner from seeing family members or friends, getting a job, or going to school.
- Keeping all the family money under one's control and/or refusing to buy food and/or necessities or pay bills.

How Teens are Affected

If there is abuse between adults or between adults and children in the home, that abuse creates the living environment of the child or teen. This environment sets the standards that teens incorporate into their social interactions and dating relationships. These patterns often repeat themselves in the families of the future. Domestic violence and the resolution of conflict through aggression and violence

leaves the teen with emotional scars that may take years to heal, and may require counseling.

Domestic violence affects people of every age and sex—every ethnic and socioeconomic group. Typically, however, the vast majority of victims are women. The abusers are typically men. Children and teens living in a home where the mother is abused are more likely to be abused or neglected by the abuser. Those who witness abuse are victims as well. The effect of domestic violence on emotional health is significant.

Where to Find Help

Victims of abuse are often reluctant to seek outside help for themselves (or their children). If your teen is a victim of abuse, the first step is to get him or her to tell *someone*: you or another trusted adult, a friend, a relative, anyone your teen believes will not blame him or her for the abuse. You should report all abuse to the police. *If your teen is in immediate danger, call 911.*

If the abuser follows your teen, makes threatening phone calls, or engages in other forms of harassment, you may be able to file for a do-it-yourself Personal Protection Order. Forms are available at your local County Clerk or Circuit Court office, or call 1-800-996-6228.

What Families Can Do

- Teach teens positive ways to handle negative emotions—anger, jealousy, sadness—and how to manage their reactions to disappointment, rejection, ridicule, peer pressure, exclusion, and conflict.

- Help teens channel or diffuse anger and other negative emotions. Teens need to understand that violence begets violence.
- Learn how to discipline your children without hitting or resorting to verbal attacks (many books are available). The use of verbal and physical abuse at home teaches that this is the way to resolve problems. Kids learn that they can control others by being abusive.
- Control access to television programs. Children and teens are vulnerable to violence and its effects. Violent movies and television shows also seem more real if the neighborhood is filled with assault or homicide.
- Limit access to guns. If your family has a gun, keep it unloaded and in a locked place. Teens and children should not be told the lock's combination or the location of the key.
- Avoid drugs and alcohol. Both substances lower inhibitions and the ability to cope with conflict. Adults are key role models.

Abusive Relationships

More and more, today's teens are finding themselves in the kind of abusive relationships that in the past have been associated with adulthood and usually marriage. The following three paragraphs explain what every adult should understand about teens and the characteristics of abusive relationships.

Violence in any relationship is never the tip of the iceberg. Violence *is* the iceberg, and any proof or sign of violence

---

Resources to Stop Violence

National helpline: 1-800-799-SAFE (1-800-799-7233).

Michigan Family Violence helpline: 1-800-99-NO-ABUSE (1-800-996-6228).

Local crisis intervention hotlines: Look in the *Yellow Pages* under Crisis Intervention, Domestic Violence, Hotlines & Help Lines (after Hotels), or Emergency Services. (You may call telephone information for these same numbers.)

---

in your teen's relationship should mean an end to that relationship, whatever it takes to accomplish that.

Adults need to clearly communicate displeasure about the violence in the relationship instead of just saying they dislike their teen's friend. Your direct verbal attack on an abuser may make your teen defensive, and make him or her want to stay in the relationship *because* you disapprove.

Adults need to step in—and step in strongly—in any instance where they believe their child is being verbally or physically abused, coerced for sex, or has become involved with another teen or young adult that is breaking the law, using drugs or alcohol, or driving drunk.

Relationship Dynamics

Abusive relationships are not always violent. Many times, the abuse takes the form of verbal, emotional, and sexual behavior designed to intimidate and control the victim. If violence does occur in the relationship, it is rarely in the beginning, and even more rarely something that will end.

As in adult relationships, males are most frequently the abuser. Families of teenage girls should be wary of boys that seem violent, excessively jealous, or show signs of abusing alcohol or drugs. That much is just common sense. You may notice behavior in other young men that simply doesn't make your daughter feel good about herself. You may need to be very direct and ask your daughter what it is that makes a person attracted to someone who makes them feel bad. Below are some more early warning signs of an abusive relationship.

- *Isolation*—Families and teens need to know that isolation—from other social activities, friends, and even family—is really the first step into an abusive relationship. The abuser seeks control, and there is no better route to control than cutting someone off from all the other things in life that would point to the fact that something is wrong with the relationship. Isolation keeps the victims of abuse silent and allows the relationship to continue.
- *Fear*—Intimidation is another key part of abusive relationships. A victim may be subjected to almost constant criticism and made to feel accountable to the abuser for every action.
- *Bruises or injuries*—As a caring adult, you have the right to ask your teen about bruises or injuries that you see. You may not get a straight answer back, which in itself should tell you something.

Your teen may also try to hide bruises with clothing—long sleeves, slacks, or turtlenecks—or sunglasses or excessive make-up. He or she may try to avoid being seen by you for several days after an abusive incident.

Stormy Relationships

Although not always violent, pay special attention if your son or daughter is involved in a relationship that is frequently stormy. The classic pattern for a battering relationship involves cycles of tension and emotional or physical "explosions," followed by apologies and attempts to win the partner back. The danger in stormy relationships is that the level of violence may increase with each succeeding cycle.

Getting Your Teen Out

The victims of abuse are usually the last to see the abuse and frequently the least able to stop the abuse. Abusers—in this sense, victims as well—are also unable or unwilling to see the relationship rationally. Your role as a parent is to put an end to the relationship and to protect your teen. To end an abusive relationship you may need to first seek help for yourself before you can help your teen. Talking with another adult you trust is always a good first step—your religious leader, your teen's counselor or school official, a crisis center counselor or someone in your state's or county's public health department. These individuals may be able to provide referrals for long-term assistance.

Use the tips below to talk with your teen, whether or not he or she is involved in an abusive relationship.

- Abuse in a relationship is a crime.
- Violence against another person is a crime.
- The abuser—not the victim—is the one at fault in abusive relationships and the one who is responsible to the legal system for criminal behavior.
- The police can and do treat abusive relationships as a crime. You or your teen can report abuse at any time.

To the Families of Young Men

Parents and other caring adults, schools, and law enforcement agencies are increasingly holding young men accountable for aggressive or violent behavior that in years past was largely considered "normal." Many families today are teaching their young children and their teens that violence is *never* the solution to a problem. If you suspect that your son is the abuser in a relationship, understand that your son needs help. The first step is putting an end to the abusive relationship. The second step is getting him some professional help.

Violence on Television

It is easy—almost fashionable—to blame television violence and violence in movies, magazines, and in the lyrics of rock music for all that is wrong with our society. There *is* something wrong with how much violence is shown on television, and violence on television *does* affect teens negatively. But as you read, consider the flip side of the equation.

Why are teens watching so much TV? What can your family do to provide alternatives to watching TV?

Frankly, the number of hours the average teen spends watching television—some 28 hours a week—is just too much, regardless of what is being shown. Those 28 hours a week are hours away from school work—especially homework—hours away from after-school activities, from part-time jobs, hours away from reading and hobbies, and hours away from being with family and friends.

The Effect of Television Violence

From the millions and millions of words spoken and written about violence on television, adults need to know a single, indisputable fact: *Overexposure to TV and movie violence increases the likelihood of aggression and violence in children and teens.*

Simply put, violence on television breeds violence and aggression in the home, at school, and on the street. Watching violence on television affects how teens view the real world, and how they respond to violence in the real world.

Teens who watch a great deal of violence on television come to see the world around them as more violent than it really is. In turn, their world view is more fearful than necessary. Such teens are more likely to see themselves as the victim of violence. Ironically, this TV-inspired world view leads to a more calloused view of real violence, whether shown as indifference to violence against others in general or an unwillingness to take action on behalf of the victim of violence in a specific incident.

Television and Your Teen

Television programs deal with many of the same issues of finding an identity that are part of normal adolescence. Issues such as sexuality, personal conflict, power, and following or not following rules are the standard fare of television programming. You can help your teen see television and television violence for what they really are.

- Set limits to TV viewing and help your teen find positive alternatives to watching TV. Most experts agree that teens should only watch about one-to-two hours of television a day.
- Watch TV with your teen. Many teens assume that television depicts realistic situations, and may become drawn into the story more than adults. Question the situations you see on TV and ask questions about how characters behave and what they do.
- Let your teen know how you feel about television violence and be prepared to take a stand on violence.

As with other issues, your influence regarding violence on TV and in movies is crucial at this time in your teen's life. You may need to make a special effort to spend time with your teen, but the effort will be worth your while.

Gangs and Violence

The police define a gang as two or more people who form an allegiance for a criminal purpose. The gang claims a geographical territory, regularly meets for criminal purposes, and uses intimidation and violence as a means for criminal purposes.

What Is Gang Graffiti?

Graffiti—inscriptions or drawings on walls or other public surfaces—is a form of vandalism classified by police as "malicious destruction of property." Gangs use graffiti to communicate. Graffiti marks gang territory, advertises the status or power of a gang, warns outsiders away from the gang's territory, and identifies individual members of a gang.

Graffiti places an economic burden both on businesses and homeowners by reducing property values. Area residents learn to fear new graffiti as a sign of potential violence in the neighborhood.

Gang graffiti can be identified by noting the symbols used. A heart, a crown, pointed stars, a sword, or a devil's horn, tail, or pitchfork are all commonly used as gang symbols. Symbols that are upside down, crossed out, or split in half are signs of disrespect or a challenge from one gang to another. The misuse of a gang's graffiti is considered very serious and can lead to violent retribution. The letter "K" following the initials of a gang member or an "X" crossing out a gang member's initials are usually a sign of violence, including homicide.

Adults should note that gang graffiti is not always found in public. Gang members, especially younger children not yet in a gang, often draw graffiti on their clothes, books, and papers from school.

Gang members show their gang allegiance in a variety of ways. Some gang members identify themselves by tilting their caps to the right or to the left or by wearing bandannas of a certain color or pattern. Other forms of showing gang ties include the placement of jewelry, the rolling of pant legs, or wearing a certain color of shoelaces. Haircuts, streaked hair, or hair worn with certain rubber bands or barrettes is another sign of gang affiliation. Some gangs alter athletic wear to match gang colors or modify the logos of brand name athletic shoes to match gang logos.

Police officers report that some young teen gang members do not dress in gang clothing or exhibit conspicuous gang behavior. Officers urge continual monitoring of teen behavior and keeping communication links between you and your teen open.

What Families Can Do

Teens join gangs to fill a void in their lives, to find things that are missing at home, in school, or in the community. The strongest reason teens give for joining a gang is "wanting to belong." Make sure your teen understands how strongly you feel about gangs.

- Stress the negative aspects of gangs at home. Point out the negative influences gangs have on individual gang members, families, neighborhoods, and the larger community. Focus on the crime, violence, and possible time in jail or prison that gang members face.
- Follow up with your teen if you see any gang graffiti or gang clothing in your home. Let your teen know how much and why you disapprove of gangs, gang graffiti, or gang clothing.

Below are a few more suggestions to help your teen "belong" to more positive groups.

- Know your teen's friends and who influences your teen.
- Know where your teen is and what he or she is doing.
- Help your teen plan constructive days and weekends. Plan family activities, especially activities where you can spend some time alone with your son or daughter.
- Encourage high academic standards, provide reading materials, and discourage excessive television viewing.
- Encourage your teen to participate in school activities.
- Volunteer at your teen's school, whether in a classroom, on a decision making or policy board, or helping out with extra-curricular activities.
- Form a personal relationship with at least one person at your teen's high school. The person you choose should have the same goals for your teen as you do.

Community Coalitions

Community coalitions formed to protect all citizens are very powerful forces for teens and against gangs. Forming a community coalition requires working with your local police. Members of the coalition should include representatives from the police, families, schools, business owners, and local government officials.

The New West Willow Neighborhood Association in Washtenaw County, Michigan, developed an extensive program of alternatives for kids in an area where gangs are pervasive. The Community Resource Center is housed in what used to be an abandoned house, and is funded solely on community contributions and volunteer efforts. The Association also works with Eastern Michigan University and Americore to provide academic tutoring after school, by appointment, five days a week. Four churches in the area work with the volunteers to provide space, services and activities, when possible.

The group puts on Halloween, Christmas, and other seasonal parties with an anti-drug/anti-gang theme. These parties are funded solely by the volunteers themselves. Working with the Recreation Department, the volunteers promote alternatives to gang activity such as softball, baseball, and soccer.

The West Willow community tries hardest to reach at-risk children who may have siblings and/or parents who have been involved in gang activities. The most reachable are elementary and middle school students. Unfortunately, these students are also the easiest to reach by gangs, and they are targeted with intimidation and violence.

The success of the New West Willow Neighborhood Association is due to the volunteers, organizations, and families who have been willing to give of time and talent to better the lives of children who are affected by and who are vulnerable to gang activities.

If you live in an area affected by gang activity and violence, don't give up. Communities working together and asking for help from business, agencies, religious organizations, and schools can offer alternatives to gang involvement.

"Domestic Violence" *reviewed by Jean Chabut, M.P.H., Chief, Center for Health Promotion and Chronic Disease Prevention, Michigan Department of Community Health, Lansing, Michigan.*

"Abusive Relationships" *contributions and review by Gloria Krys, M.A., C.S.W., L.P.C., Program Coordinator, Assault Crisis Center of Washtenaw County Community Mental Health (1866 Packard Road, Ypsilanti, Michigan 48197. 24-hour Crisis line: 313-483-7273).*

"Domestic Violence" and "Abusive Relationships" *reviewed by Mr. Jan Christensen, J.D., M.S.W., Chief, Division of Violence, Injury, and Surveillance, Center for Health Promotion and Chronic Disease Prevention, Community Public Health Agency, Lansing, Michigan, and*

Patricia Smith, M.S., Violence Prevention Program, Center for Health Promotion and Chronic Disease Prevention, Community Public Health Agency, Lansing, Michigan.

"Gangs and Family Action" *contributions by Detective Sergeants Larry Ivory and Michael Oliver, Waterford Township Police Department, Waterford, Michigan.*

Reviewed by Sergeant Darwin A. Scott, Criminal Intelligence Unit, Michigan Department of State Police, East Lansing, Michigan.

New West Willow Neighborhood Association project from Bob Talbert, Detroit Free Press Columnist (March 7, 1996), and a telephone interview with Lt. Mike Radzik at the Washtenaw County Sheriff's Department (March 13, 1996).

Chapter 14

TEENS AND A BETTER COMMUNITY

Framework for Success

Behind the headlines about youth violence, crime, pregnancy, and other problems, is an even more important and urgent story: In all towns and cities across America, the developmental infrastructure is crumbling.

Too few young people grow up experiencing key ingredients for their healthy development. They do not experience support from adults, build relationships across generations, or hear consistent messages about boundaries and values. Most have too little to do that is positive and constructive. The result is that communities and the nation are overwhelmed with problems and needs in the lives of youth.

Thus, the real challenge facing America is not to attack one problem at a time in a desperate attempt to stop the hemorrhaging. The real challenge is to rebuild the developmental infrastructure for our children and adolescents.

Though the professionals and the public sector have a role to play, much of the responsibility and capacity for the healthy development of youth is in the hands of the people. Search Institute, located in Minneapolis, Minnesota, has created a model for understanding the developmental needs of children and adolescents. Rooted in research on more than 250,000 American youth in grades six to twelve, the framework identifies forty building blocks, or "developmental assets," that all children and adolescents need to grow up healthy, competent, and caring (see

"Appendix A"). These assets provide a powerful paradigm for mobilizing communities, organizations, and individuals to take action for youth—action that can make a real difference.

The Power of Assets

When drawn together, these forty developmental assets are powerful shapers of young people's behavior. The more assets young people experience, the more they engage in positive behaviors, such as volunteering and succeeding in school. The fewer assets kids have, the more likely they are to engage in risk-taking behaviors, violent acts, and other negative behaviors. Thus, while each asset must be understood and is important, the most powerful message of developmental assets comes in seeing all forty as a whole. These assets are cumulative—the more the better.

In short, young people who experience more of these assets are more likely to grow up caring, competent, and responsible. This important relationship between developmental assets and choices made has been documented for all types of youth, regardless of age, gender, geographical region, town size, or race/ethnicity.

The Crumbling Infrastructure

Most people recognize that influences such as caring families, discipline, educational commitments, social skills, and other assets are important for healthy development. Yet society seems to have forgotten how to make sure young people experience and develop these things. Out of 250,000 students in grades six through twelve who have been surveyed, the average young person experiences only about sixteen of the forty assets. Furthermore, 76 percent of young people experience twenty or fewer assets.

The "asset gap" exists in all types and sizes of communities. In fact, youth in 95 percent of the communities studied to date report an average of fifteen to seventeen assets. Thus, in virtually every town, suburb, and city in America, far too many young people are struggling to construct their lives without an adequate foundation upon which to build.

What has happened? Many of the ways society has provided these assets are no longer in place because of major societal changes: Most adults no longer consider it their responsibility to play a role in the lives of children outside their nuclear family. Also, parents are less available for their children because of demands outside the home and cultural norms that undervalue parenting. Non-family adults, and institutions have become uncomfortable articulating values or enforcing appropriate boundaries for behavior.

Over the past twenty-five years, American society has become more and more age-segregated, providing fewer opportunities for meaningful inter-generational relationships. Socializing systems (families, schools, congregations, etc.) have become more isolated, competitive, and suspicious of each other.

In place of the extended family/caring community, the mass media have become influential shapers of young people's attitudes, norms, and values. As problems—and solutions—have become more complex, more of the responsibility for young people has been turned over to professionals.

The Healthy Community

For several decades, Americans have invested tremendous time, energy, and resources in trying to combat symptoms of these changes. It hasn't worked. It is time for a new approach—an approach that focuses energy, creativity, and resources into rebuilding the developmental foundation for all youth.

As we begin shifting our thinking, we can anticipate creating communities where all young people are valued and valuable, problems are more manageable, and an attitude of vision, hope, and celebration pervades community life.

Based on literature, research, and work with numerous communities, Search Institute has begun developing a list of key characteristics of healthy communities for youth. The list follows.

Community Mindset:
- Children and youth are a top priority.
- All citizens have responsibility for children and youth.
- All citizens have pro-child power.
- Community understands that all children need more assets.
- Emphasis is placed on building family strengths.
- The community "wraps its arms" around teenagers.
- Community balances prevention and promotion.

Community Data:
- Community has gathered good data on pro-child resources, programs, and strategies.

- Community understands levels of assets and at-risk behaviors in its own youth, and monitors changes in assets and at-risk behaviors.

Community Norms:
- The community shares and demonstrates in concrete ways basic values such as responsibility, respect, honesty, justice, and equality.
- Community has clear and consistent policies on alcohol and other drugs that are consistently and actively put into practice.

Community Programming:
- After-school care is available for all children and youth.
- There is a rich variety of school-based, community, and religious organizations that involve most youth in constructive activities.
- Organizations have expansive missions that include both prevention and promotion.
- Youth programs operate with a partnership mentality.

- Programs reinforce each other with appropriate redundancy.
- Peers educate and support each other.
- Mentoring is widespread (youth to youth, and adult to youth).
- Young people are involved in and empowered through community service.

Community Education:
- Parent education is available, and parents participate in it.
- Adult volunteers receive training and continuing education.
- Schools are caring and supportive for youth.

Collaboration:
- Community cooperation and collaboration occurs effectively across multiple sectors.

Reprinted with permission from Healthy Communities: Healthy Youth: A National Initiative of Search Institute to Unite Communities for Children and Adolescents, *by Eugene C. Roehlkepartain and Peter L. Benson (Search Institute, Minneapolis, MN: 1996). All rights reserved by Search Institute, 1-800-888-7828.*

Search Institute's 40 Developmental Assets for Youth

(Based on surveys of more than 250,000 youth in 450 communities across the United States.)

EXTERNAL ASSETS

Support

1. **Family Support**—Family life provides high levels of love and support.
2. **Positive family communication**—Young person and her or his parent(s) communicate positively, and young person is willing to seek parent(s') advice and counsel.
3. **Other adult relationships**—Young person receives support from three or more non-parent adults.
4. **Caring neighborhood**—Young person experiences caring neighbors.
5. **Caring school climate**—School provides a caring, encouraging environment.
6. **Parent involvement in schooling**—Parent(s) are involved in helping youth succeed in school.

Empowerment

7. **Community values youth**—Young person perceives that adults in the community value youth.
8. **Youth as resources**—Young people are given useful roles in the community.
9. **Service to others**—Young person serves in the community one hour or more per week.
10. **Safety**—Young person feels safe at home, school, and in the neighborhood.

Boundaries and Expectations

11. **Family boundaries**—Family has clear rules and consequences, and monitors the young person's whereabouts.
12. **School boundaries**—School provides clear rules and consequences.
13. **Neighborhood boundaries**—Neighbors take responsibility for monitoring young people's behavior.
14. **Adult role models**—Parent(s) and other adults model positive, responsible behavior.
15. **Positive peer influence**—Young person's best friends model responsible behavior.
16. **High expectations**—Both parent(s) and teachers encourage the young person to do well.

Constructive Use of Time

17. **Creative activities**—Young person spends three or more hours per week in lessons or practice in music.
18. **Youth programs**—Young person spends three or more hours per week in sports, clubs, or organizations at school and/or in community organizations.
19. **Religious community**—Young person spends one or more hours per week in activities in a religious institution.
20. **Time at home**—Young person is out with friends "with nothing special to do" two or fewer nights per week.

INTERNAL ASSETS

Commitment to Learning

21. *Achievement motivation*—Young person is motivated to do well in school.
22. *School engagement*—Young person is actively engaged in learning.
23. *Homework*—Young person reports doing at least one hour of homework every school day.
24. *Bonding to school*—Young person cares about his or her school.
25. *Reading for pleasure*—Young person reads for pleasure three or more hours per week.

Positive Values

26. *Caring*—Young person places high value on helping other people.
27. *Equality and social justice*—Young person places high value on promoting equality and reducing hunger and poverty.
28. *Integrity*—Young person acts on convictions and stands up for her or his beliefs.
29. *Honesty*—Young person tells the truth even when it is not easy.
30. *Responsibility*—Young person accepts and takes personal responsibility.
31. *Restraint*—Young person believes it is important not to be sexually active or to use alcohol or other drugs.

Social Competencies

32. *Planning and decision-making*—Young person knows how to plan ahead and make choices.
33. *Interpersonal competence*—Young person has empathy, sensitivity, and friendship skills.
34. *Cultural competence*—Young person has knowledge of and comfort with people of different cultural/racial/ethnic backgrounds.
35. *Resistance skills*—Young person can resist negative peer pressure and dangerous situations.
36. *Peaceful conflict resolution*—Young person seeks to resolve conflict non-violently.

Positive Identity

37. *Personal power*—Young person feels he or she has control over "things that happen to me."
38. *Self-esteem*—Young person reports having a high self-esteem.
39. *Sense of power*—Young person reports that "my life has a purpose."
40. *Positive view of personal future*—Young person is optimistic about her or his personal future.

From Peter L. Benson, *Creating Healthy Communities for Children and Adolescents* (Jossey-Bass, San Francisco, CA, 1996). For more information about fostering these assets in youth and involving communities, call the Search Institute at 1-800-888-7828.

5 Things Families Can Do to Build Assets

1. Post the list of 30 assets on your refrigerator door. Each day, purposefully nurture at least one asset.

2. Model—and talk about—the values and priorities you wish to pass on to your children.

3. Take time to nurture your own assets by spending time with supportive people, using your time constructively, and reflecting on your own values and commitments.

4. Regularly do things with your child, including projects around the house, recreational activities, and service projects.

5. Talk to your children about assets. Ask them for suggestions of ways to strengthen assets.

5 Things Adults Can Do to Build Assets

1. Look at and greet every child or adolescent you see.

2. Have a five-minute conversation with a child or adolescent about her or his interests.

3. Send a "thinking of you" or birthday card, letter, or e-mail message to a child or teen.

4. Invite a young person to do something you enjoy doing together (play a game, go to a park, go to a movie, etc.).

5. Have an open-door policy in your neighborhood so kids feel welcome in your home for refreshments, conversation, or just hanging out.

5 Things You Can Do to Mobilize Your Community for Asset Building

1. Talk with leaders, friends, neighbors, and other citizens about the vision and potential for asset building. Share materials that describe the asset-building approach.

2. Sponsor community-wide or regional events to talk about asset building and its potential. Invite influential people to the event. Also work hard to include youth, parents, senior citizens, and other people.

3. Gather information on what's currently happening in your community and how it could be enhanced with an asset-building focus or partnership.

4. Work with a cross-section of leaders and other citizens to develop plans or strategies for an asset-building initiative.

5. Serve on a committee or task force to implement asset-building strategies.

The Impact of Developmental Assets

Based on Search Institute's study of more than 250,000 youth across the nation, this chart shows that the more assets young people experience, the less likely they are to engage in a wide range of risky behaviors. In addition, youth with more assets are more likely to grow up doing the positive things that society values.

Number of Assets a Teen Has →	1-10 Assets	11-20 Assets	21-25 Assets	26-30 Assets	National Average
Positive Behavior					
Volunteer Service	15%	34%	57%	75%	37%
(One or more hours per week)					
Success in School	5%	13%	28%	51%	18%
(Get mostly A's in school)					
Risk-Taking Behavior					
Alcohol Use	44%	23%	9%	3%	22%
(6 or more uses in the past month or got drunk once or more in past two weeks)					
Sexual Activity	51%	34%	17%	7%	32%
(Sexual intercourse, two or more times in life)					
Violence/Anti Social Activity	51%	28%	13%	5%	28%
(Two or more acts in the past year)					
School Trouble	30%	12%	4%	1%	13%
(Skipped school two or more days in the past month and/or wants to drop out)					

Appendix B

Table 1: Epstein's Framework of Six Types of Involvement and Sample Practices

Type 1 Parenting	Type 2 Communicating	Type 3 Volunteering	Type 4 Learning at Home	Type 5 Decision Making	Type 6 Collaborating with Community
Help all families establish home environments to support children as students.	Design effective forms of school-to-home and home-to-school communications about school programs and children's progress.	Recruit and organize parent help and support.	Provide information and ideas to families about how to help students at home with homework and other curriculum-related activities, decisions, and planning.	Include parents in school decisions, developing parent leaders and representatives.	Identify and integrate resources and services from the community to strengthen school programs, family practices, and student learning and development.
Sample Practices	**Sample Practices**	**Sample Practices**	**Sample Practices**	**Sample Practices**	**Sample Practices**
Suggestions for home conditions that support learning at each grade level. Workshops, videotapes, computerized phone messages on parenting and child rearing at each age and grade level. Parent education and other courses or training for parents (e.g., GED, college, credit, family literacy). Family support programs to assist families with health, nutrition, and other services. Home visits at transition points to preschool, elementary, middle, and high school. Neighborhood meetings to help families understand schools and to help schools understand families.	Conferences with every parent at least once a year, with follow-ups as needed. Language translators to assist families as needed. Weekly or monthly folders of student work sent home for review and comments. Parent/student pickup of report card, with conferences on improving grades. Regular schedule of useful notices, memos, phone calls, newsletters, and other communications. Clear information on choosing schools or courses, programs, and activities within schools. Clear information on all school policies, programs, reforms, and transitions.	School and classroom volunteer program to help teachers, administrators, students, and other parents. Parent room or family center for volunteer work, meetings, resources for families. Annual postcard survey to identify all available talent, times, and locations of volunteers. Class parent, telephone tree, or other structures to provide all families with needed information. Parent patrols or other activities to aid safety and operation of school programs.	Information for families on skills required for students in all subjects at each grade. Information on homework policies and how to monitor and discuss schoolwork at home. Information on how to assist students to improve skills on various class and school assessments. Regular schedule of homework that requires students to discuss and interact with families on what they are learning in class. Calendars with activities for parents and students at home. Family math, science, and reading activities at school. Summer learning packets or activities. Family participation in setting student goals each year and in planning for college or work.	Active PTA/PTO or other parent organizations, advisory councils, or committees (e.g., curriculum, safety, personnel) for parent leadership and participation. Independent advocacy groups to lobby and work for school reform and improvements. District-level councils and committees for family and community involvement. Information on school or local elections for school representatives. Networks to link all families with parent representatives.	Information for students and families on community health, cultural, recreational, social support, and other programs or services. Information on community activities that link to learning skills and talents, including summer programs for students. Service integration through partnerships involving school; civic, counseling, cultural, health, recreation, and other agencies and organizations; and businesses. Service to the community by students, families, and schools (e.g., music, drams, and other activities for seniors or others). Participation of alumni in school programs for students.

Tables 1, 2 and 3 printed with special permission, Phi Delta Kappan, May 1995. School/Family/Community Partnership, Caring for the Children We Share (p. 701-711) by Joyce L. Epstein. Additional information on parent involvement will appear in Joyce Epstein's forthcoming book, School and Family Partnerships: Preparing Educators and Improving Schools, to be published by Westview Press, Boulder, CO. Contact Dr. Epstein at The Center on Families, Communities, Schools and Children's Learning, Johns Hopkins University, 3505 N. Charles St., Baltimore, MD 21218 or call (410) 516-8800.

Table 2: Epstein's Challenges and Redefinitions for the Six Types of Involvement					
Type 1 Parenting	Type 2 Communicating	Type 3 Volunteering	Type 4 Learning at Home	Type 5 Decision Making	Type 6 Collaborating with Community
Challenges	**Challenges**	**Challenges**	**Challenges**	**Challenges**	**Challenges**
Provide information to *all* families who want it or who need it, not just to the few who can attend workshops or meetings at the school building. Enable families to share information with schools about culture, background, children's talents and needs. Make sure that all information for and from families is clear, usable, and linked to children's success in school.	Review the readability, clarity, form, and frequency of all memos, notices, and other print and non-print communications. Consider parents who do not speak English well, do not read well, or need large type. Review the quality of major communications (newsletters, report cards, conference schedules, and so on). Establish clear two-way channels for communications from home to school and from school to home.	Recruit volunteers widely so that *all* families know that their time and talents are welcome. Make flexible schedules for volunteers, assemblies, and events to enable parents who work to participate. Organize volunteer work; provide training; match time and talent with school, teacher, and student needs; and recognize efforts so that participants are productive.	Design and organize a regular schedule of interactive homework (e.g., weekly or bimonthly) that gives *students* responsibility for discussing important things they are learning and helps families stay aware of the content of their children's classwork. Coordinate family-linked homework activities, if students have several teachers. Involve families and their children in all important curriculum-related decisions.	Include parent leaders from all racial, ethnic, socioeconomic, and other groups in the school. Offer training to enable leaders to serve as representatives of other families, with input from and return of information to all parents. Include students (along with parents) in decision-making groups.	Solve turf problems of responsibilities, funds, staff, and locations for collaborative activities. Inform families of community programs for students, such as mentoring, tutoring, business partnerships. Assure equity of opportunities for students and families to participate in community programs or to obtain services. Match community contributions with school goals; integrate child and family services with education.
Redefinitions	**Redefinitions**	**Redefinitions**	**Redefinitions**	**Redefinitions**	**Redefinitions**
"Workshop" to mean more than a *meeting* about a topic held at the school building at a particular time. "Workshop" may also mean making information about a topic available in a variety of forms that can be viewed, heard, or read anywhere, any time, in varied forms.	"Communications about school programs and student progress" to mean two-way, three-way, and many-way channels of communication that connect schools, families, students, and the community.	"Volunteer" to mean anyone who supports school goals and children's learning or development in any way, at any place, and at any time—not just during the school day and at the school building.	"Homework" to mean not only work done alone, but also interactive activities shared with others at home or in the community, linking schoolwork to real life. "Help" at home to mean encouraging, listening, reacting, praising, guiding, monitoring, and discussing—not "teaching" school subjects.	"Decision making" to mean a process of partnership, of shared views and actions toward shared goals, not just a power struggle between conflicting ideas. Parent "leader" to mean a real representative, with opportunities and support to hear from and communicate with other families.	"Community" to mean not only the neighborhoods where students' homes and schools are located but also any neighborhoods that influence their learning and development. "Community" rated not only by low or high social or economic qualities, but by strengths and talents to support students, families, and schools. "Community" means all who are interested in and affected by the quality of education, not just those with children in the schools.

Table 3: Epstein's Expected Results of the Six Types of Involvement for Students, Parents, and Teachers

Type 1 Parenting	Type 2 Communicating	Type 3 Volunteering	Type 4 Learning at Home	Type 5 Decision Making	Type 6 Collaborating with Community
Results for Students	Results for Students	Results for Students	Results for Students	Results for Students	Results for Students
Awareness of family supervision; respect for parents. Positive personal qualities, habits, beliefs, and values, as taught by family. Balance between time spent on chores, on other activities, and on homework. Good or improved attendance. Awareness of importance of school.	Awareness of own progress and of actions needed to maintain or improve grades. Understanding of school policies on behavior, attendance, and other areas of student conduct. Informed decisions about courses and programs. Awareness of own role in partnerships, serving as courier and communicator.	Skill in communicating with adults. Increased learning of skills that receive tutoring or targeted attention from volunteers. Awareness of many skills, talents, occupations, and contributions of parents and other volunteers.	Gains in skills, abilities, and test scores linked to homework and classwork. Homework completion. Positive attitude toward schoolwork. View of parent as more similar to teacher and of home as more similar to school. Self-concept of ability as learner.	Awareness of representation of families in school decisions. Understanding that student rights are protected. Specific benefits linked to policies enacted by parent organizations and experienced by students.	Increased skills and talents through enriched curricular and extracurricular experiences. Awareness of careers and of options for future education and work. Specific benefits linked to programs, services, resources, and opportunities that connect students with community.
For Parents	For Parents	For Parents	For Parents	For Parents	For Parents
Understanding of and confidence about parenting, child and adolescent development, and changes in home conditions for learning as children proceed through school. Awareness of own and others' challenges in parenting. Feeling of support from school and other parents.	Understanding school programs and policies. Monitoring and awareness of child's progress. Responding effectively to students' problems. Interactions with teachers and ease of communication with school and teachers.	Understanding teacher's job, increased comfort in school, and carry-over of school activities at home. Self-confidence about ability to work in school and with children or to take steps to improve own education. Awareness that families are welcome and valued at school. Gains in specific skills of volunteer work.	Know how to support, encourage, and help student at home each year. Discussions of school, classwork, and homework. Understanding of instructional program each year and of what child is learning in each subject. Appreciation of teaching skills. Awareness of child as a learner.	Input into policies that affect child's education. Feeling of ownership of school. Awareness of parents' voices in school decisions. Shared experiences and connections with other families. Awareness of school, district, and state policies.	Knowledge and use of local resources by family and child to increase skills and talents or to obtain needed services. Interactions with other families in community activities. Awareness of school's role in the community and of community's contributions to the school.
For Teachers	For Teachers	For Teachers	For Teachers	For Teachers	For Teachers
Understanding families' backgrounds, cultures, concerns, goals, needs, and views of their children. Respect for families' strengths and efforts. Understanding of student diversity. Awareness of own skills to share information on child development.	Increased diversity and use of communications with families and awareness of own ability to communicate clearly. Appreciation for and use of parent network for communications. Increased ability to elicit and understand family views on children's programs and progress.	Readiness to involve families in new ways, including those who do not volunteer at school. Awareness of parents' talents and interests in school and children. Greater individual attention to students, with help from volunteers.	Better design of homework assignments. Respect of family time. Recognition of equal helpfulness of single-parent, dual-income, and less formally educated families in motivating and reinforcing student learning. Satisfaction with family involvement and support.	Awareness of parent perspectives as a factor in policy development and decisions. View of equal status of family representatives on committees and in leadership roles.	Awareness of community resources to enrich curriculum and instruction. Openness to and skill in using mentors, business partners, community volunteers, and others to assist students and augment teaching practice. Knowledgeable, helpful referrals of children and families to needed services.

Appendix C

Table 4: Michigan Laws Relating to Substances: Use, Possession, Delivery, Selling, and Furnishing—1996

ALCOHOL	
Under Age 21 Blood Alcohol Content (BAC) of .02 percent to .07 percent	
First Offense	$250 fine + costs 30-60 day license suspension* (restrictions allowed) Up to 45 days community service 4 points added to license
Second Offense	Up to $500 fine + costs 90 days to 1 year license suspension* Up to 60 days community service
Minors in Possession of Alcohol (17-20 years)	
First Offense	Up to $100 fine, possible community service, possible alcohol screening.
Second Offense	Up to $200 fine 90-180 day license suspension*
Third Offense	Up to $500 fine 180 days to 1 year license suspension*
Attempt to purchase or to consume alcohol (under 21)	
First Offense	Up to $100 fine, possible community service, possible substance abuse screening
Second Offense	Up to $200 fine, may be ordered to participate in substance abuse treatment, possible community service, possible license restrictions/suspension*
Third Offense	Up to $500 fine, may be ordered to participate in substance abuse treatment, possible community service, possible license restrictions/suspension*
Open intoxicants in a motor vehicle (misdemeanor)	Up to $100 fine; up to 90 days in jail Violators under 17 years of age petitioned to Juvenile Court
License reinstatement fee is $125 when driving privileges are returned.	
TOBACCO	
Use or possession by minors under age 18 in any public place (civil infraction)	Up to $50 fine In school or on school grounds: $50 fine State law is misdemeanor with a $50 fine
MARIJUANA	
Possession (misdemeanor)	Up to 1 year, $2,000 fine, or both
Delivery (felony):	
1. Less than 5 kilograms <u>or</u> fewer than 20 plants	Up to 4 years and/or up to $2,000 fine
2. Five kilograms or more (but less than 45 kgm) <u>or</u> 20 plants or more (but fewer than 200 plants)	Up to 7 years and/or up to $500,000 fine
3. 45 kgm or more <u>or</u> 200 plants or more	Up to 15 years and/or up to $10 million fine

COCAINE	
Possession (felony)	
1. 25 grams or under	Up to 4 years and/or up to $25,000 fine
2. Greater than 25 grams (but not more than 50 grams)	Mandatory 1-4 year or life probation <u>and</u> up to $25,000 fine
2. Greater than 50 grams (but not more than 225 grams)	Mandatory 10-20 years
3. Greater than 225 grams (but not more than 650 grams)	Mandatory 20-30 years
4. 650 grams or more	Mandatory life sentence

The Law and Adults

In addition to the laws affecting teens listed above, parents and guardians should be aware that Michigan laws regarding controlled substances affect them, as responsible adults. In summary:

- A person who knowingly sells or furnishes alcohol to a person who is less than 21 years of age, or who fails to make diligent inquiry as to whether the person is less than 21 years of age, is guilty of a misdemeanor.

- A person who violates this law shall be fined $1,000 and may be sentenced to imprisonment for up to 60 days for a first offense, shall be fined $2,500 and shall be sentenced to imprisonment for up to 90 days for a second or subsequent offense, and may be ordered to perform community service.

- If the subsequent consumption of the alcohol by the person less than 21 years of age is a direct and substantial cause of that person's death or an accidental injury that causes that person's death, a person who violates this subsection is guilty of a felony, punishable by imprisonment for not more than 10 years, or a fine of not more than $5,000 or both,

Local laws affecting controlled substances vary. In general, adults are responsible for whatever happens on their own property. A person who knowingly allows consumption of alcohol and the use of other, illegal substances is subject to penalties, fines, and possible imprisonment. Please become aware of such laws in your area, and inform your teen of all laws that affect them, their friends, and you.

Contributions and review by:

Detective Ronald Halcrow of the Birmingham Police Department, Birmingham, Michigan.

The Michigan Department of State Police: Sergeant Joseph Hanley, Special Operations, Traffic Services Division; Lt. Dan Smith of the Traffic Services Division; and Phyllis Good, Supervisor of the Narcotics and Dangerous Drugs Unit, East Lansing Laboratory, East Lansing, Michigan.

Appendix D

Admissions Requirements for Michigan's Public Universities

The state universities of Michigan have adopted specific admissions requirements for students seeking regular admission to a four-year degree program. These requirements are explained in detail in a document developed by the Presidents Council, State Universities of Michigan, entitled *Designing Your Future*, which provides students with guidance in selecting courses to enhance their preparation for university level work. Copies of *Designing Your Future* are available through your school's guidance counselor.

The public universities have agreed that, to be eligible for regular admission, students must successfully complete the following course of study during high school:

- *English*—four years required.
- *Mathematics*—three years required, including intermediate algebra; four years strongly recommended.
- *Biological/Physical Sciences*—two years required; three years strongly recommended; to include one year of biological science and one year of physical science. At least one year of a laboratory course is also strongly recommended.
- *History* and *Social Sciences*—three years required; one year of American history and one year of world history strongly recommended.

Prospective students are also encouraged to complete courses in the following areas:

- *Foreign Language*—three years strongly recommended.
- *Fine and Performing Arts*—two years strongly recommended.
- *Computer Literacy*—one year of hands-on experience in using computers strongly recommended.

The universities recognize that, for a variety of reasons, some students may not be able to complete all of the requirements. In such circumstances, students may be considered for admission and, therefore, are encouraged to apply to the university of their choice. In all instances, each university has final authority for admissions decisions, based on the level of achievement required and other indicators of potential for academic success.

Students are encouraged to make the best use of courses that are offered at their high school. By doing so, they are more likely to develop the competencies and skills that are essential for academic success and, at the same time, have greater control over their choice of college and career options.

From the Presidents Council, State Universities of Michigan, 230 N. Washington Square, Suite 302, Lansing, Michigan 48933 (517-482-1563), March 1991. (Information is accurate in February 1997).

Resources

For help locating all types of services for families and individuals in the Detroit and Tri-County areas, and for a free, wallet-sized reference card of area service agencies for you and your teen, call *Tel-Help*, a United Way Community Services Agency, at 1-800-552-1183 or 313-226-9888 in Detroit.

COLLEGE, SCHOOL, AND WORK

College Guides

America's Best Colleges, U.S. News and World Report (U.S. News Specialty Marketing, Department 300M, P.O. Box 2284, South Burlington, VT 05407-2284; 1996, $5.95 plus $4.00 for shipping/handling).

Barron's Top 50: An Inside Look at America's Best Colleges, Barron's (1996, $14.95). Reviews by recent graduates of colleges. Describes academic programs, admissions, financial aid, social life, and extracurricular activities.

Barron's Compact Guide to Colleges (10th Edition), Barron's (1996, $8.95). Lists and describes 400 well-known schools across the U.S.

Competitive Colleges: Top Colleges for Top Students - 1996-1997, Peterson's ($16.95). Profiles more than 375 leading colleges.

Fiske Guide to Colleges 1997 (New York Times Books, 1996, $19.00).

The Insider's Guide to Colleges, Staff of Yale Daily News (St. Martin's Griffin, 1996, $14.99).

A National Directory of Four-Year Colleges, Two-Year Colleges, and Post-High School Training Programs for Young People with Learning Disabilities, P.M. Fielding (Partners in Publishing, 1992, $29.95).

Peterson's Four-Year Colleges 1997 (Peterson's, 1997, $21.95). Peterson's also produces specialty guides, such as *Top Colleges for Science* and *Handbook for College Admissions*.

Profiles of American Colleges: Northeast (12th Edition), The Editors of Barron's Educational Series, Inc. (1996, $13.95). Presents complete college listings and descriptions from twelve northeastern states: CT, DE, DC, ME, MD, MA, RI, NH, NJ, NY, PA, VT.

Financial Aid for College

Don't Miss Out: The Ambitious Student's Guide to Financial Aid, Joseph Re (Octameron Associates, P.O. Box 2748, Alexandria, VA 22301 or call 1-703-836-5480, 1995, $9.50). Excellent guide to college aid.

The Financial Aid Book details over 194,000 financial aid opportunities ($19.95) and *The Government Financial Aid Book* gives an inside look at state and federal grants and loans (revised by Perpetual Press, 1996, $9.95; 1-800-807-3030 or contact http://ReadersNdex.com/perpetual).

The 5 W's of Financial Aid (Michigan Higher Education Assistance Authority; Support Services Program, Office of Student Financial Aid, P.O. Box 30466, Lansing, Michigan 48909-7966). This book also includes information on federal programs.

How to Pay for College: A Practical Guide to Getting the Money You Need (video and guidebook), John Spiropoulos (Information Video, Inc., 9115 Crosby Road, Silver Spring, MD 20910 or call 301-587-1984; $29.95 + shipping & handling; 1989). Parents how-to on applying for financial aid. Very thorough and easy to understand.

The Student Guide (U.S. Department of Education; 1-800-433-3243; Federal Student Aid Information Center, P.O. Box 84, Washington, DC 20044-0084).

Financial Aid Web Sites

Fastweb: http://www.studentservices.com/Fastweb for a free, searchable database of more than 180,000 private sector scholarships, grants, and loans.

Financial Aid Information Page: http://www.finaid.org for an aid estimator and scholarship service scam alerts by Mark Kantrowitz, author of the *Prentice Hall Guide to Scholarships and Fellowships for Math and Science Students* (Prentice Hall, 1993, $19.95).

Kaplan Student Loan Information Program: http://www.kaploan.com for free, downloadable software to help families estimate their share of college costs.

National Association for College Admission Counseling Fair: Call 703-836-2222 or contact www.nacac.com. Metro Detroit Fair is April 15,

1997: contact 810-348-5600 for details. For western U.S. fairs, contact the **Rocky Mountain Association for College Admission Counseling** fairs at 505-835-5424.

U.S. Department of Education: http://easi.ed. gov for information on federal aid programs and to file their Free Application for Federal Student Aid via *FAFSA Express.*

School and Work Success

Clicking: 16 Trends to Future Fit Your Life, Your Work, and Your Business, Faith Popcorn (HarperCollins, 1996, $26.00). Shows how trends can be used to put your professional and personal lives in synch with the future.

College Freshman Survival Guide, John Spiropoulos (Information Video, Inc., 9115 Crosby Road, Silver Spring, MD 20910 or call 301-587-1984; $29.95 + shipping & handling; 1992). Good video on the difficulties faced by first-year college students. Advice from older students and freshman.

Family Life and School Achievement: Why Poor Black Children Succeed or Fail, Reginald M. Clark, Ph.D. (available through the Center for Improvement of Child Caring, Studio City, California; 1-800-325-CICC, $14.95). Compares the backgrounds of high achieving inner city teenagers with peers who are failing, and determines what makes the difference.

The Gifted Kids Survival Guide: A Teen Handbook, Judy Galbraith, M.A., and Jim Delisle, Ph.D. (Free Spirit Publishing, 1996, $14.95). New facts, findings, and insights about giftedness, intelligence testing, and IQ; school survival, success, and learning; goal-setting, planning for the future, and college preparation.

How to Become a SuperStar Student, Professor Tom McGee of Worland High School (video: 1995, $39.95 + $5.00 shipping/handling). Tom McGee's lectures build the foundation of achievement that can last a lifetime. Reading for results, writing without pain, studying to succeed, and organizing your time. Packed with information.

How to Prepare for SAT I, Samuel Brownstein, Mitchel Weiner, and Sharon Weiner Green (*Barron's SAT I Manual*, 19th Ed., 1997, $16.95) and *How to Prepare for the ACT* by George Ehrenshaft, Robert L. Lehrman, Fred Obrecht, and Allan Mundsack (*Barron's ACT Manual*, 10th

Ed. plus a Computer Disk, February 1995, $29.95). Test prep manual plus a computer disk containing one full-length practice test and extra drill and review questions.

Imagine the Future: A Teenager's Guide to the Next Century and Beyond and *Parent's Guide— Imagine the Future: Helping Your Teen Prepare for the Future*, Joseph Malgeri (Career Solutions, 1997, $8.95 each or $15.95 for the set; quantity discounts available; 810-879-0681). These books will awaken, challenge, and motivate teens and parents to take control of the future now.

Preparing Students for the 21st Century, Donna Uchida with Marvin Cetron and Floretta McKenzie (American Association of School Administrators, 1996, $14.95). What families and schools can do help prepare teens for success in the 21st century.

Student Success Secrets, by Eric Jensen, illustrated by Tom Kerr (Barron's Educational Series, Inc., 1996, $8.95). Sure-fire study strategies that can increase test scores and raise grades dramatically. Advice on developing motivation to learn. Good-humored and approachable style (cartoons included).

Teaching the New Basic Skills: Principles for Educating Children to Thrive in a Changing Economy, Frank Levy and Richard J. Murane (Free Press, 1996, $24.00). Drawing on the work of real teachers, parents, and administrators, this book provides a blueprint for turning our schools around.

What Kids Need to Succeed, Peter L. Benson, Judy Galbraith, and Pamela Espeland (Search Institute, 1995; 1-800-888-7828; $4.99 + $3.50 shipping/handling). More than 500 common-sense ideas for building assets in youth.

What Smart Students Know, Adam Robinson (Crown Publishers Inc., 1993, $16.00). Contains hundreds of practical tips about "maximum grades, optimum learning, minimum time."

The Winner-Take-All Society, Robert H. Frank and Philip J. Cook (The Free Press, 1995). An analysis of "Winner-Take-All" markets and the jobs that are created and won by the elite.

DEPRESSION AND TEEN SUICIDE

Conversations at The Carter Center: Coping with the Stigma of Mental Illness (video), hosted by Rosalynn Carter; narrated by Joanne Woodward (27 minutes; The Carter Center Mental Health Program, One Copenhill, Atlanta, GA 30307; 404-420-5165; $7.00: requests for free copies considered). Author Kathy Cronkite and actor Rod Steiger discuss their personal experiences coping with mental illness and then answer questions from a live audience. Treatments are discussed.

Helping Your Depressed Teenager: A Guide for Parents and Caregivers, Gerald D. Oster, Ph.D., and Sarah S. Montgomery, M.S.W. (John Wiley & Sons, 1994, $23.95). Covers teen development, understanding depression, and how to help your teen.

How to Cope with Depression—A Complete Guide for You and Your Family, J. Raymond DePaulo Jr., M.D., and Keith R. Ablow, M.D. (Ballantine Books, 1996, $10.00). Depression from four perspectives: Disease, personality, behavior, and life stories.

Journey: A Story for Survivors, Pamela Quay Farlow-Wolgast (booklet, 1978, $3.50; 810-456-0909). Inspirational reading for people who have lost someone to suicide.

Life Happens: A Teenager's Guide to Friends, Failure, Sexuality, Love, Rejection, Addition, Peer Pressure, Families, Loss, Depression, and Change, Charles Wibbelsman, M.D., and Kathy McCoy (Perigee, 1996, $11.00).

No One Saw My Pain: Why Teens Kill Themselves, Andrew Slaby, M.D., and Lili Frank Garfinkel (W.W. Norton & Company, 1994, $12.00). Slaby, a psychiatrist specializing in depression and crisis intervention, found that the severity of distress in teens was missed because people didn't know what to look for.

Now We Can Successfully Treat the Illness Called Depression, National Foundation for Depressive Illness, Inc. (P.O. Box 2257 New York, NY 10116; 800-248-4344; free). Defines depressive illnesses and describes treatment options. Other booklets available.

Suicide: Why? Adina Wrobleski (Afterwords, 1995, $12.95) Features 85 questions and answers about suicide.

Depression/Suicide Resources

American Suicide Foundation: 212-410-1111, 1045 Park Avenue, New York, NY 10028.

Common Ground 24-Hour Crisis Line: 800-231-1127 or 810-456-0909. Helps callers or links them to one of 4,500 resources nationwide.

Depression and Related Affective Disorders Association (DRADA): 410-955-4647. Local chapters and help.

Mental Health Association of Michigan: 800-482-9534. Referrals, brochures, support groups, and other information and advocacy.

National Alliance for the Mentally Ill: 703-524-7600. Local chapters.

National Foundation for Depressive Illness, Inc.: 800-245-4305. Information and a list of physicians who specialize in affective disorders.

National Institutes of Mental Health: 800-421-4211. Offers free brochures on depression.

National Depressive and Manic Depressive Association: 312-642-0049. Offers mail-order bookstore on depression. For a free catalog, write: NDMDA, 730 N. Franklin, Suite 501, Chicago, IL 60610.

Recovery Inc.: 312-337-5661. Self-help group to identify self-defeating and illness promoting thoughts and impulses and replace them with self-endorsing thoughts and actions. For a group near you, send a S.A.S.E. to 802 N. Dearborn St., Chicago, IL 60610.

Suicide Prevention Center: Emergency Telephone Service 313-224-7000. Referral to nearest crisis center.

Suicide Prevention Resources: 212-750-8410. Help line (347 East 61 Street, Room 1-RE, New York, NY 10021).

Learning Differences Resources

CHAADD (Children and Adults with Attention Deficit Disorders): 800-233-4050. Parents/professionals: How to organize support groups, information on conferences and chapters.

Council for Exceptional Children; Eric Clearinghouse on Disabilities and Gifted Children: 800-328-0272

Learning Disabilities Association of America: 517-485-8160. Free materials and referrals (500 chapters).

In Michigan:
ADHD Lifespan Center: 313-745-4882. For all ages. Diagnosis, psychological testing and therapy, education, medication, and school advocacy. (Wayne State Univ/Detroit Medical Ctr/Children's Hospital).

Beaumont Center for Human Development: 810-691-4744, 8 a.m. to 5 p.m. weekdays. Evaluation services, tutoring, and counseling (Royal Oak).

Crittenton Hospital Psychiatric Evaluation Referral Center: 810-652-5797. Open 24 hours (Rochester).

Eton Transition Center: 810-642-1150, 8 a.m. to 4:30 p.m. weekdays. Individualized curriculum for learning disabled students (Birmingham, Michigan).

Michigan Association for Children and Adults with Learning Disabilities: 517-485-8160, 8 a.m. to 1 p.m. weekdays. Student advocacy, parent support, conferences, and addresses of local chapters.

Michigan Dyslexia Institute, Inc.: 1-800-832-3535 or 517-485-4000. Six centers statewide. Testing, instruction, conferences, teacher training, summer camp, materials store (1-800-495-6758).

University Psychiatric Centers (WSU): Diagnosis and treatment for ADHD.
Children's Hospital, Detroit	313-745-4892
Southfield/Cranbrook	810-540-2545
Commerce Township	810-360-4005
Warren	810-558-8900
Livonia	313-464-4220
Southfield/Oakland	810-352-9570
Jefferson Avenue, Detroit	313-993-3434

Understanding Depression: A Complete Guide to Its Diagnosis & Treatment, Donald F. Klein, M.D. and Paul H. Wender, M.D. (Oxford University Press, 1993, $16.95). A definitive guide to depressive illness—its causes, course, and symptoms.

LEARNING DIFFERENCES

Attention Deficit Disorder Association: 8091 South Ireland Way, Aurora, CO 80016; 303-690-7548.

Attention Deficit Disorder Warehouse: 1-800-233-9273. Many of the following books are available.

Dyslexia Store, Michigan Dyslexia Institute/Dyslexia Association of America, 532 E. Shiawassee Street, Lansing, MI 48912-1214: 1-800-495-6758, 517-485-4076 fax. Carries extensive line of books on dyslexia and learning disabilities (free catalog).

National Center for Learning Disabilities, 381 Park Avenue South, Suite 1420, New York, NY 10016; 212-545-7510

National Dyslexia Research Foundation, 333 Park Avenue, P.O. Box 393, Boca Grande, FL 33921; 1-800-424-READ.

1100 Words You Need to Know, Murray Bromberg and Melvin Gordon (Barron's Educational Series, 1993, $10.95). A 46-week program to increase critical, commonly used vocabulary. Good for dyslexia: Excellent preparation for ACT and SAT tests and college-level reading.

1995-1996 Directory of Facilities and Services for the Learning Disabled (16th edition: Academic Therapy Publications, 20 Commercial Blvd, Novato, CA 94949-6191). Copies available at no charge; requests should include a $4 postage/handling fee for each copy. $12 postage/handling for 5 copies. Volume discounts available.

About Dyslexia: Unraveling The Myth, Priscilla Vail (Modern Learning Press, 1990, $10.00). A book of insight into the strengths and weaknesses of people with dyslexia.

ADHD and Teens: A Parent's Guide to Making It Through the Tough Years, Colleen Alexander-Roberts (Taylor Publishing, 1995, $13.00). Teens with ADHD have an extremely high risk of school and social problems which can lead to academic failure and disruptive family relationships. Practical advice.

Attention Deficit Disorder: A Different Perception, Thom Hartmann (Underwood Books, 1993, $10.95). Provides an inside view of how people with ADD think and function in society.

Driven to Distraction: Recognizing and Coping with Attention Deficit Disorder from Childhood through Adulthood, Edward M. Hallowell, M.D., John J. Ratey, M.D. (Pantheon Books, 1994, $13.00). Readable, useful book on ADHD. Stories from child and adult sufferers.

Dyslexia: Background for an Action Agenda for Teacher Training, John C. Howell, Ph.D. (available at the Dyslexia Store, 1-800-495-6758 or 517-485-4076 fax, $5.00). A must read for teachers, school administrators, and parents. Clear, concise, and compelling, Dr. Howell answers your questions regarding dyslexia.

Help for the Learning Disabled Child: Symptoms and Solutions, Lou Stewart, M.A.T./L.D. (Slosson Educational Publications, 1-800-828-4800, 1990, $29.95). Aid to parents and professionals. Confirms learning disabled (LD) and ADHD symptoms and provides methods to use.

A Layman's Look at Dyslexia, Ronald E. Weger (available at the Dyslexia Store, 1-800-495-6758 or 517-485-4076 fax, $10.00). Covers dyslexia from statistics to individual triumphs. Easy reading.

Living with a Learning Disability, Barbara Cordoni (Southern Illinois University Press, 1991, $15.95). Social barriers can cause more of a loss of self esteem and personal pain than academic proficiency.

A National Directory of Four-Year Colleges, Two-Year Colleges, and Post-High School Training Programs for Young People with Learning Disabilities, P.M. Fielding (Partners in Publishing, 1992, $29.95).

The Survival Guide for Teenagers with LD (Learning Differences), Rhoda Cummings, Ed.D., and Gary Fisher, Ph.D. (Free Spirit Publishing, 1996, $11.95 + shipping/handling; audio tape available for $19.95). Clear, comprehensive, and matter-of-fact, this guide helps teens with LD succeed in school and prepare for life as adults.

Surviving Public School: A Guide for Parents of Learning Disabled (Dyslexic) Kids, Thomas W. Conwell (available at the Dyslexia Store, 1-800-495-6758 or 517-485-4076 fax, $10.00). A step-by-step plan for not only surviving public school, but winning the war for your child.

Taking Charge of ADHD, Russell A. Barkley, Ph.D. (Guilford Press, New York, 1995, $16.95). Provides the most comprehensive, up-to-date information and expert advice on managing children and adolescents with ADHD.

Teenagers with ADD: A Parents' Guide, Chris A. Ziegler Dendy, M.S. (Woodbine House, 1995, $18.95). Gives parents necessary tools to raise a healthy teen with positive attitudes.

What Every Teacher and Parent Should Know About Dyslexia, Dave Sargent and Laura Tirella (Ozark Publishing, 1995, $29.95). Questions and answers, suggestions for parents and modifications for teachers.

PHYSICAL HEALTH

Cookbooks

Heart Smart® Cookbook, Henry Ford Heart and Vascular Institute and The Detroit Free Press (Detroit Free Press©, 1991, $14.95; 1-800-245-5082). Simple suggestions and recipes to help you cut saturated fats and promote a healthier lifestyle.

High Fit—Low Fat Cookbook and *High Fit—Low Fat Vegetarian Cookbook*, Lizzie Burt, I.A.C.P. et. al. (The University of Michigan Medical Center, P.O. Box 363, Ann Arbor, Michigan 48106-0363; 1-800-433-MFIT: $14.95 + $4.00 shipping/handling 1st book, $1.00 s/h each additional book). If you think healthy recipes are boring, these books will change your mind.

The New Laurel's Kitchen: A Handbook for Vegetarian Cookery and Nutrition, Carol Flinders, Brian Ruppenthal, and Laurel Robertson (Ten-Speed Press, 1996, $29.95).

Moosewood Restaurant Low-Fat Favorites, The Moosewood Collective (Clarkston Potter, 1996, $22.00: available through CSPI Holiday Fare, Suite 300, 1875 Connecticut Ave., N.W., Washington, DC 20009-5728; 1-800-237-4874). More than 250 low-fat recipes for homey, hearty food. Except for chapter on fish, most recipes are vegetarian.

Nutrition and Health Resources

American Anorexia/Bulimia Association, Inc. (AABA): 212-501-8351, 9 a.m. to 5 p.m. weekdays. Information on eating disorders, referrals to clinics, hospital programs and support groups.

American Diabetes Association: 1-800-342-2383. 8:30 a.m. to 5 p.m. EST weekdays. Brochures & referrals.

The American Dietetic Association Consumer Nutrition Hotline: 1-800-366-1655. 10 a.m. to 5 p.m. EST weekdays. Speak to dietitians, referrals, and publications.

American Heart Association: 1-800-432-7854. 8:30 a.m. to 4:30 p.m. EST weekdays. Brochures & information.

Anorexia Nervosa and Related Eating Disorders, Inc. (ANRED): 503-344-1144 (P.O. Box 5102, Eugene, Oregon 97405).

Food Allergy Network: 1-800-929-4040, or send a SASE to 4744 Holly Avenue, Fairfax, VA 22030. Publisher of brochures & bimonthly newsletter.

National Association of Anorexia Nervosa and Associated Disorders (ANAD): 847-831-3438, 9 a.m. to 5 p.m. weekdays. Free information, telephone counseling and nationwide referrals to therapists, support groups, and physicians.

National Cancer Institute: 1-800-422-6237. 9 a.m. to 7 p.m. EST weekdays. Publications, approved mammography facilities, speak to cancer specialists.

USDA Meat and Poultry Hotline: 1-800-535-4555 (Washington DC residents call 202-720-3333). 10 a.m. to 4 p.m. EST weekdays. Food safety.

The Wellness Encyclopedia of Food and Nutrition, Sheldon Margen, M.D. (Random House, 1992, $35.00). One of the most authoritative guides to shopping and eating for better health and longer life. See also *The Simply Healthy Lowfat Cookbook, The Wellness Lowfat Cookbook*, with Dale A. Ogar.

Eating Disorders (free); *Eating for Life* ($1.00); *Food Allergies: Rare but Risky* (free); *Should You Go On a Diet?* (for teens—free). Write to R. Woods, Consumer Information Center - 6A-2, P.O. Box 100, Pueblo, Colorado 81002 for these publications and/or a complete catalog of available publications. Internet Web address: http://www.-gsa.gov/ staff/pa/cic/cic.htm.

Eating Habits and Disorders, Rachel Epstein (Chelsea House Publishers, New York; Encyclopedia of Health; 1990, $19.95). Comprehensive information about basic biology, preventive medicine, and medical and surgical treatments—to be healthy throughout life.

The Food Guide Pyramid (Home and Garden Bulletin #252, U.S. Department of Agriculture, 6505 Belcrest Road, Hyattsville, MD 20782). Send stamped, self-addressed envelope.

The Healthy Eaters Guide to Family & Chain Restaurants: What to Eat in Over 100 Restaurant Chains across America, Hope S. Warshaw, M.M.Sc., R.D. (Chronimed Publishing, 1993, $9.95). Shows which foods are the healthiest in more than 100 of the most popular family and chain restaurants in America.

Hunger Pains: The Modern Woman's Tragic Quest for Thinness, Mary Pipher (Ballantine Books, 1997, $10.00). From the author of *Reviving Ophelia*.

The MFit Grocery Shopping Guide: Your Guide to Healthier Choices!, Nelda Mercer, M.S., R.D., Lori Mosca, M.D., M.P.H., and Melvyn Rubenfire, M.D. (Favorite Recipes Press, 1995, $18.95; 1-800-433-MFIT). Total guide to which foods are the best for you. Over 10,000 brand name foods.

A Parent's Guide to Anorexia and Bulimia, Katherine Byrne (Henry Holt, 1989, $9.95) Sympathetic support and positive advice for families. How to handle everyday problems and evaluate treatment options. Based on the author's personal experience with her daughter.

Presidential Sports Award: We Challenge You and *Get Fit: A Handbook for Youth Ages 6-17* and *Physical Education: A Performance Checklist,* (President's Council on Physical Fitness and Sports, Washington, DC, 20004). Three free booklets.

Real Gorgeous: The Truth About Body & Beauty, Kaz Kooke (W.W. Norton, New York, 1996, $13.00). A good, hard look at how girls and women have been mislead to think they should look like a model. Kaz Kooke uses her great sense of humor, funny chapter titles, and illustrations to make her point: each of us is special in her own way. Good reading for boys and men, as well.

Total Nutrition: The Only Guide You'll Ever Need from the Mt. Sinai School of Medicine, Victor Herbert, M.D., J.D., and Genell J. Subak-Sharpe, M.S., Editors (St. Martin's Griffin, 1995, $16.95). An easy-to-read, thorough, all-in-one reference book for average people—an educated approach to healthy eating.

SCHOOL-FAMILY-COMMUNITY PARTNERSHIPS

Beyond the Classroom: Why School Reform has Failed and What Parents Need to Do, Laurence Steinberg, Bradford Brown, and Sanford M. Dornbusch (Simon & Schuster, 1996). By the time teenagers reach high school, peer influence outweighs parental influence. More kids feared negative reactions from peers for high grades than negative reactions from parents for low grades. Authors list suggestions for parents. Critics say this is the most important book on this subject in 10 years.

Breaking Ranks: Changing an American Institution, National Association of Secondary School Principals (1904 Association Drive, Reston, VA 22091-1537; 1-800-253-7746; 1996, $19.50 + $3.00 shipping/handling). The report of the Association in partnership with the Carnegie Foundation for the Advancement of Teaching on the high school of the 21st century.

1) Building Assets in Youth (video), Peter L. Benson (1995; $24.95 + $4.50 shipping/-handling). 12-minute video describes the power of asset building in youth. Includes a leader's guide. *2) Healthy Communities: Healthy Youth*, Eugene C. Roehlkepartain and Peter L. Benson (1996; free). Individuals, families, and communities taking responsibility to foster asset-building in youth for a better future. Very inspiring. *3) Uniting Communities for Youth*, Dr. Peter L. Benson (1995; free). Focuses on how communities can work to develop positive assets in youth. For a catalog of these and other Search Institute publications, call 1-800-888-7828.

Innovations in Parent and Family Involvement, J. William Rioux and Nancy Berla (Eye on Education Inc., P.O. Box 388, Princeton Junction, NJ 08550, 1993). Leading advocates of parent involvement write a definitive book; Chapter Five gives examples of successful programs in high schools. Strategies and tips for those who want their program to work.

Matter of Time: Risk and Opportunity in the Out-of-School Hours, (Carnegie Council on Adolescent Development, Carnegie Corporation of New York, 1994). A partnership needs to look at school use after formal school hours. An extraordinary booklet.

The New American Family and the School, J. Howard Johnston (National Middle School Association, 4807 Evanswood Dr., Columbus, OH 43229, 1990, $6.00). Frank, to-the-point; be sure to read the chapter on barriers to home-school cooperation.

The Scapegoat Generation: America's War on Adolescents, Mike A. Males (Common Courage Press, P.O. Box 702, Monroe, Maine 04951, 1996, $17.95). A must-read for anyone interested in redefining both modern adolescence and the challenge faced by all Americans to ensure the next generation's future.

Strong Families, Strong Schools: Building Community Partnerships for Learning (U.S. Dept. of Education, 600 Independence Ave. S.W., Washington, DC 20202; call 1-800-USA-LEARN to obtain a free copy). Be sure to send for this 50-page, well designed booklet with the most important message you could read: "How important families and communities are to the success of our children in school."

Schools/Family/Community Partnerships: Caring for the Children We Share, Joyce L. Epstein (*Phi Delta Kappan,* May 1995, p. 701-712). Describes the reasons for developing partnerships and five important steps to activating a plan. Extensive bibliography. Important; check at your library.

Taking Stock: Views of Teachers, Parents and Students on School, Family, and Community Partnerships in High Schools, Lori J. Conners and Joyce L. Epstein. (Report No. 25, 1994 Center on Families, Communities, Schools and Children's Learning, The Johns Hopkins University, 3505 N. Charles St., Baltimore, MD 21218;

410-516-8800.) A report on the successes of six high schools deeply involved in *Action Teams* to promote family involvement.

"The 10th School: Where School-Family-Community Partnerships Flourish," Don Davies (*Education Week*, July 10, 1996). Exactly what can be done to make your school the 1 out of 10 in which collaboration between teachers and administrators and families and communities is commonplace. Worth a trip to the library, or ask your principal for a copy.

SEXUAL ABUSE

Abused Boys: The Neglected Victims of Sexual Abuse, Mic Hunter (Fawcett Columbine, 1990, $10) Dispels myths and misinformation, and offers an overview for recovery.

Basic Facts About Child Sexual Abuse (National Committee for Prevention of Child Abuse, P.O. Box 94283, Chicago, IL 60690; 800-835-2671; Order #702480, $4.75) Answers basic questions about abuse. Also publishes a free catalog.

Two books from KIDSRIGHTS by Catalina Herrerias, M.S.W., Ph.D.: *Parent Talk: A Parent's Guide to Child Sexual Abuse Prevention* (1993, $4.95); and *Teen to Teen: Personal Safety and Sexual Abuse Prevention* (1996, $4.95) This second book is written especially for teens. Straight talk, attractive; easy to read material every teen must understand. Call KIDSRIGHTS at 1-800-892-5437.

The Survivor's Guide: For Teenage Girls Surviving Sexual Abuse, Sharice A. Lee, (Sage Publications, 1995, $12.95). Common effects of sexual abuse on the survivor; encourages the survivor to seek help and introduces the concept of recovery. Helps the reader to cease blaming herself. Real examples of adolescents' experiences regarding the effects of sexual abuse.

SEXUAL ISSUES

My Body, My Self, Lynda Madaras and Area Madaras (Newmarket Press, 18 East 48th Street, New York, NY 10017, 212-832-3575; 1993; $9.95). Illustrations, quizzes, and exercises for preteen and teenage girls exploring the physical changes of puberty.

How to Talk with Your Teenagers About the Facts of Life, Planned Parenthood Federation of America, Inc. (Marketing Department, 810 7th

---

Sexual Abuse: Finding Help

Anyone who suspects a child is being exploited by an adult, sexually or otherwise, should contact the local police department. Children 15 and under cannot legally consent to an act of sexual penetration, and children 12 and under cannot consent to any sexual contact, according to Nancy Diehl, director of the child and family abuse bureau of the Wayne County Prosecutor's Office, Detroit, Michigan.

The Michigan Family Independence Agency (former Department of Social Services) funds the Runaway Assistance Program, which provides referrals and crisis intervention for runaway children and their parents. The 24-hour hot line number is 1-800-292-4517. The Agency also offers a 24-hour Parent Helpline, 1-800-942-4357, for parents who need counseling or a referral.

Contact your local Child Protective Services, listed under State of Michigan, or your own state's government listings.

Ave., New York, NY 10010; 1-800-669-0156; or call a local office; 1995, $3.00). Straight answers to most-asked questions about puberty, reproduction, pregnancy, contraception, and sexuality.

Period, (Revised with a removable Parent's Guide) J. Gardner-Loulan, B. Lopez; M. Quackenbush (Volcano Press, P.O. Box 270, Volcano, CA 95689; 209-296-3445, 1993, $9.95 + $4.50 shipping) National Science Teacher's Association says, "this is perhaps the only satisfactory book on this important topic."

Raising Sexually-Healthy Children, Lynn Leight (Avon Books, 105 Madison Avenue, New York, NY 10016, 1990, $10) A guide for parents on talking with children and teens about sexuality, STDs, AIDS and other topics.

Talking with Your Child About Sex (Item B-114) and *Talking with Your Teen About Sex* (Item B-115) (To receive a catalog, please send $1.00 to cover postage and handling to: National PTA, 135 S. LaSalle St., Dept. 1860, Chicago, IL 60674-1860; or call (312) 5493253).

The What's Happening to My Body Book for Girls, and The What's Happening to My Body Book for Boys, Lynda Madaras (Newmarket Press, 18 East 48th Street, New York, NY 10017,

212-832-3575: 1987; $9.95) Written for parents and their daughters and sons, this is a guide to the changes of puberty, along with information on AIDS, sexually transmitted disease, and birth control.

Sexually Transmitted Diseases (STD's)

The following publications can be purchased from Health Education Services, A Division of Health Research Inc., P.O. Box 7126, Albany, NY 12224; 518-439-7286. Catalog available. The first two publications below are in full- color, comic book format, and easy-to-read, but contain explicit graphics and subject matter—with story lines on avoiding AIDS. All three are published by the State of New York Department of Health.

- *A Close Encounter* (1988, 14 pp., 75¢).
- *Flirting With Danger* (1994, 16 pp., 75¢).
- *What Parents Need to Tell Children About AIDS* (1992, 10 pp. booklet, 75¢).

AIDS Answers for Teens, Linda Schwartz (The Learning Works, Inc., P.O. Box 6187, Santa Barbara, CA 93160, 1993; $5.95). Factual information about AIDS. Written specifically for teens in grades 7-12. Good home resource.

AIDS-Proofing Your Kids: A Step-by-Step Guide, Loren Acker, Bram Goldwater, William Dyson (Beyond Words Publishing, Inc., 13950 NW Pumpkin Ridge Rd., Hillsboro, OR 97124, 503-647-5109, $7.95, 1992) A how-to book for parents and teachers about helping teenagers avoid HIV/-AIDS.

Common Questions About AIDS and HIV Infection (Michigan Department of Community Health, Community Public Health Agency, HIV/AIDS Prevention & Intervention Section; P.O. Box 30035, Lansing, MI 48909; 517-335-8371; 1993, free).

Deciding About Sex: The Choice to Abstain (#138) and *STD Facts* (#153, or #165 in Spanish) (Network Publications, P.O. Box 1830, Santa Cruz, CA 95061-1830; 1-800- 321-4407; send self-addressed, stamped envelope with 65 cents postage for up to five free pamphlets).

The Family Heart: A Memoir of When Our Son Came Out, Robb Forman Dew (Addison-Wesley, 1994, $11.00 paperback). Dew takes the reader on a journey of acceptance as she deals with the fact that her son is gay. She shows readers understanding far beyond tolerance.

STD Information & Help

For more information or to speak to someone about sexually transmitted disease, you may call the Centers for Disease Control (CDC) National Hot Lines:

CDC National AIDS Hotline:
1-800-342-2437 (always open)
Spanish 1-800-344-7432

CDC National STD Hotline:
1-800-227-8922, 8 a.m. to 11 p.m. EST weekdays.

Herpes Resource Center:
1-800-230-6039, 9 a.m. to 7 p.m. EST weekdays

The National AIDS Hotline:
1-800-342-AIDS, 24 hours;
1-800-344-7432, Spanish;
1-800-243-7889, TDD, TTY.
Provides referrals to local AIDS organizations as well as general information and education.

National AIDS Clearinghouse:
1-800-458-5231.

Clinical Trials:
1-800-TRIALS-A (1-800-874-2572)
9 a.m. to 7 p.m. weekdays.
Source of the National Institutes of Allergy and Infectious Diseases. Offers latest on all AIDS studies.

State of Michigan Hotline:
1-800-872-AIDS (1-800-872-2437)
TDD 1-800-332-0849.

Series: *How to Help Yourself: 1) Taking the HIV(AIDS) Test; 2) Testing Positive for HIV; 3) Infections Linked to AIDS; 4) The Lung Infection; 5) The Brain Infection; 6) HIV- Related TB; 7) AIDS-Related MAC.* (U.S. Department of Health and Human Services, Public Health Service, National Institute of Health, Bethesda, MD 20892. Call 1-800-458-5231 for free copies.)

Talking With Kids About AIDS - Teaching Guide and Resource Manual, Jennifer Tiffany, Donald Tobias, and others (Cornell University Resource Center, 7 Business and Technology Park, Ithaca, NY 14850; 607-255-2080; 1993; $10.75 includes shipping). Step-by-step illustrated explanations of what HIV/AIDS is, myths, facts, and prevention. Age-appropriate sample conversations.

Yo! This Brochure is a Rap About AIDS (Detroit Urban League, 208 Mack, Detroit, MI 48201; 313-863-0300, ext. 225; free).

Parents, Families and Friends of Lesbians and Gays (PFLAG) provides support services for families and caregivers of all people with AIDS, gay or straight. Callers will be referred to volunteers in their area. Call 202-638-4200, Monday-Friday, 9:00 a.m. to 5:00 p.m.

SUBSTANCE ABUSE

Alcohol: Chemistry & Culture, Kevin R. Scheel (WRS Publishing, 701 N. New Road, Waco, TX 76710, 1994, $3.95). Outstanding booklet with extremely thorough coverage of all aspects of alcohol consumption including the physical and emotional aspects of use.

Alcohol is a Drug, Too: What Happens to Kids When We're Afraid to Say No, David Wilmes (Johnson Institute, 1993, $5.95). You will find excellent advice here.

Alcoholism at Time of Diagnosis and 29 other videos related to health: Time Life Medical (Patient Education Media, Inc., Time Life Building, 1271 6th Avenue, New York, NY 10020; 1996, $19.95). Available at video and retail stores. Excellent health videos with personal workbook/diaries and resources.

Breaking the Cycle of Addiction: A Parent's Guide to Raising Healthy Kids, Patricia O'Gorman and Philip O. Diaz (Health Communications, 1987, $8.95) Advice for parents who were raised by addicted parents. Roles of child, adults, and school in recovery, and associated problems and issues.

Children of Alcoholics: Selected Readings, Hover Adger Jr. and seven others (National Association for Children of Alcoholics, 1996). Authors among the most distinguished clinicians and researchers in the family addiction field.

Directory of Michigan Substance Abuse Programs (1996, free) and *Michigan Parent Handbook* (1996, 25¢), Michigan Resource Center (111 West Edgewood Blvd., Suite 11, Lansing, Michigan 48911; 1-800-626-4636 for materials; add shipping for orders outside Michigan). Excellent resource.

Help for Substance Abuse

Al-Anon and Alateen: 1-800-356-9996 (P.O. Box 862, Midtown Station, New York, NY 10018-0862).

Al-Anon Family Group: 1-800-344-2666. Location of meetings near you.

Alcoholics Anonymous National Referral Hotline: 1-800-252-6465 24 hours a day. Referral to local AA, Al-Anon, Nar-Anon and Al-Ateen inpatient and outpatient services.

American Council on Alcoholism: 1-800-527-5344 (2522 St. Paul Street, Baltimore, MD 21218).

American Lung Association of Michigan: 1-800-LUNG. Information on stop-smoking programs. Call 1-800-678-5864 for materials and videos.

National Association for Children of Alcoholics: 1-888-554-2627 (help line), or 301-468-0985;nacoa@prevline.health.org email address. Conferences, information, advocacy.

National Clearinghouse for Alcohol and Drug Information: 1-800-729-6686 or 301-468-2600 (P.O. Box 2345, Rockville, MD 20847-2345). Publications and videos.

National Council on Alcoholism and Drug Dependence: 1-800-NCA-CALL 8:30 a.m. to 4:30 p.m. EST. In Michigan, 1-800-344-3400. Information and referrals.

Tel-Awareness Line: 1-800-227-7209. (Brighton Hospital, Brighton, MI) Recorded messages 24 hours a day about alcohol and other drugs.

For a complete list of books and associations for children of alcoholics, send $1.00 and a SASE to Bridge Communications, Inc., 1450 Pilgrim Road, Birmingham, MI 48009.

Drinking: A Love Story, Caroline Knapp (The Dial Press/Dell Publishing, 1996, $22.95). The author's personal experience with alcoholism—and her conclusion that an alcoholic's body responds differently to liquor than a non-alcoholic's body.

Getting Your Kids to Say "No" in the '90s When You Said "Yes" in the '60s, Victor Strasburger, M.D. (Simon & Schuster, 1993, $11.00). Practical suggestions for telling your children the truth about substance abuse and teenage sex from a specialist in adolescence.

Parenting for Prevention, David Wilmes (Johnson Institute, 1989, $9.95). Individual copies free from Miller Family Foundation, Box 831463, Stone Mountain, GA 30083. Highly recommended.

Playing It Straight—Personal Conversations on Recovery, Transformation and Success, David Dodd (Health Communications, 1996, $12.95). Interviews with celebrities recovering from substance abuse and addiction whose sole purpose is to help others.

Straight Talk: A Magazine for Teens (The Learning Partnership, P.O. Box 199, Pleasantville, NY 10570-0199; 914-769-0055; $11.80 for 4-part series). Hard-hitting, to the point publication for teens on HIV/AIDS, self-esteem, substance abuse, and teen relationships. Quantity discounts available for schools.

Terry: My Daughter's Life-and-Death Struggle With Alcoholism, George McGovern (Villard/Random House, 1996, $21.00). The heart-rending story of Terry McGovern's long fight to escape alcoholism, and her untimely death.

Tips for Teens About: Marijuana; Alcohol; Smoking; Inhalants; Crack-Cocaine; Hallucinogens (Michigan Resource Center, 111 West Edgewood Blvd., Suite 11, Lansing, MI 48911, 517-882-9955 or 800-626-4636). One page front and back fliers. Write for a **Video Catalog** with 22 pages of video listings related to Alcohol, Tobacco and Other Drugs and related subjects. Videos are free to borrow. Free Action Kit that covers "every aspect of designing, planning and implementing a community based prevention effort" is available.

Trackman Presents: Facts About Drugs (video), Michigan Association For Deaf, Hearing and Speech Services (MADHS) (1-800-YOUR-EAR).

TEEN DEVELOPMENT

Before It's Too Late: Why Some Kids Get Into Trouble and What Parents Can Do About It, Stanton E. Samenow, Ph.D. (Times Books, 1989; 1-800-733-3000, $22.50 + $4.00 ship-

ping/handling). Insights into the personalities of children with problem behavior—offers practical suggestions for taking action now.

Beyond Leaf Raking: Learning to Serve/Serving to Learn, Peter L. Benson and Eugene C. Roehlkepartain (Abingdon Press, Nashville, 1993, $11.95 + $4.50 s/h). Youth who serve others are more likely to have a positive outlook on life, and are far less likely than other youth to be involved in at-risk behaviors. Practical checklists, worksheets, and surveys included.

Caring for Your Adolescent, Ages 12-21 (The American Academy of Pediatrics: Division of Publications, 141 Northwest Point Blvd., P.O. Box 927, Elk Grove Village, IL, 60009-0927; 800-433-9016; 1992; $24.50) Editorial direction by a distinguished pediatrician; contributions by 30 specialists in adolescent medicine. Complete reference guide to developmental stages and issues facing adolescents. Highly recommended.

Discipline: A Sourcebook of 50 Failsafe Techniques for Parents, James Windell (Collier Books, New York; 1991; $10.00). A psychologist for the juvenile court offers practical tips for parents to build self-control in children of all ages.

Effective Black Parenting: A Review and Synthesis of Black Perspectives, Kerby T. Alvy, Ph.D. (available through the Center for Improvement of Child Caring, Studio City, California; 1-800-325-CICC, $14.95). A complete profile of effective black parenting based on what black scholars like James Comer and Alvin Poussaint believe are the most important issues and challenges confronting black families today.

Emotional Intelligence, Daniel Goleman (Bantam Books, 1995, $23.95). Fascinating and challenging book grounded in recent scientific research. Not an easy read, but well worth the effort. Emotional intelligence includes self-awareness, impulse control, diligence, social skills, and empathy.

Every Family Needs a C.E.O., Dr. Reuben Bar-Levav (Fathering Inc. Press, 1995, $19.95). A psychiatrist for 30 years is encouraging to fathers and single mothers. He says to raise responsible children, some person must be in charge.

Family Life and School Achievement: Why Poor Black Children Succeed or Fail, Reginald M. Clark, Ph.D. (available through the Center for Improvement of Child Caring, Studio City,

California; 1-800-325-CICC, $14.95). Compares the backgrounds of high achieving inner city teenagers with peers who are failing, and determines what makes the difference.

Get it? Got it. Good!: A Guide for Teenagers, Carol Noël (Serious Business, Inc., Petoskey, Michigan, 1996, $7.95). This outstanding book for teens covers self esteem, college, working, depression, decision-making, sex, AIDS, healthy eating, crime, alcohol, smoking, and substance abuse.

Get Out of My Life: But First Could You Drive Me and Cheryl to the Mall?, Anthony E. Wolf, Ph.D. (The Noonday Press, 1995, $10.00). About adolescence—explained with quotes from kids and their families, and chapters on what they do and why, and a multitude of other issues of great concern to adults with teens. All written with humor.

Grounded for Life?! Stop Blowing Your Fuse and Start Communicating With Your Teenager, Louise Felton Tracy, M.S. (Parenting Press, Inc., 1994, $12.95) Chapters include: Begin by Changing Yourself, Natural Consequences, Parent-Owned Problems, Love in Action, Resistance and Acceptance, Understanding Teen Sexuality, Parental Persistence.

Growing Up Adopted, Peter L. Benson, Dr. Anu Sharma, L.P., and Eugene C. Roehlkepartain (Search Institute, 1995; 1-800-888-7828; $19.95 + $4.50 shipping/handling). Detailed information on the findings of Search Institute's study of adopted teens and their families.

How to Become a SuperStar Student, Professor Tom McGee of Worland High School (video: 1995, $39.95 + $5.00 shipping/handling). Tom McGee's lectures build the foundation of achievement that can last a lifetime. Reading for results, writing without pain, studying to succeed, and organizing your time. Packed with information.

Life on the Edge, James C. Dobson (Word Publishing, 1995, $15.99). For older adolescents (ages 16-26) and their parents, Dobson suggests ways to approach the life-altering decisions of college, marriage, and family.

Older, But NOT OLD ENOUGH: Families InTouch Book Six - A Book for People Ages 11-15 on Love & Sex, Alcohol, Other Drugs & AIDS, and ***Staying in Touch: Families InTouch Book Five - For Parents of Children ages 11-15***,

Joanne Barbara Koch (The Parents InTouch Project, 1991, $20.00 + $3.00 shipping/handling). Outstanding resources for families and teens.

The Parenting Tight-Rope: A Flexible Approach to Building Self-Esteem, Julie Stitt (Momentum Books, 1994, $9.95). Stitt, the prevention specialist at Common Ground, a leading crisis center in Michigan, bases her book on experience with teens.

Parenting With a Purpose: A Positive Approach for Raising Confident, Caring Youth, Dean Feldmeyer and Eugene C. Roehlkepartain (Search Institute, 1995, free; 1-800-888-7828). 14-page, full color booklet on ways families can build assets in young people. Positive and inspiring.

Parenting Your Teenager in the 1990s, David Elkind (Ballantine Books, 1994, $10.00). Explains the "whys" behind teens' emotions and behavior, and offers parents suggestions for coping with issues such as friends, family, dating, school, and society.

Parents and Adolescents Living Together, Part 1: The Basics, *and* ***Parents and Adolescents Living Together, Part 2: Family Problem Solving***, Gerald Patterson and Marion Forgatch (Castalia Publishing; 1987; Part 1: $11.95, Part 2: $12.95) Part 1: Step-by-step approach to handling arguments and conflicts between parents and teens. Part 2: Negotiation skills for resolving difficult issues.

Peer Pressure Reversal: An Adult Guide to Developing a Responsible Child, Sharon Scott (Human Resource Development Press, 1-800-822-2801 outside Maryland, or 413-253-3488 in Maryland, 1985, $9.95 + $5.00 shipping/-handling). Provides parents with a step-by-step approach to teaching how to handle peer pressure.

Raising A Son: Parents and the Making of a Healthy Man, Don Elium and Jeanne Elium (Beyond Words Publishing, 1-800-284-9673, 1992, $11.95) This book can be extremely helpful in guiding mothers and fathers as well as single parents in raising a son. Excellent bibliography included.

Reviving Ophelia: Saving the Selves of Adolescent Girls, Mary Bray Pipher (Ballantine Books, 1995, $12.95). A must-read for parents of teenage daughters. The book explains why, in spite of the women's liberation movement, girls today have a harder time growing up than ever before due to our media-dominated culture.

The 6 Vital Ingredients of Self-Esteem and How to Develop Them in Your Child, Bettie B. Youngs, Ph.D. (Rawson Associates/Macmillan Publishing Co., 1991, $22.95). A leading educator presents a step-by-step handbook for parents to help build strong positive self-esteem.

Stress and Your Child: Know the Signs and Prevent Harm, Dr. Archibald D. Hart (Word Inc., 1994, $5.99). Hart writes in a most humane and practical way about how to reduce harmful stress. Good material on discipline.

Strong Mothers, Strong Sons, Ann P. Caron (HarperPerrenial, 1995, $14.00). A book for mothers that focuses on the special needs of male adolescents, including the conflict of violence vs. sensitivity, athletics, sexuality, and attitudes toward women.

Teaching the New Basic Skills: Principles for Educating Children to Thrive in a Changing Economy, Frank Levy and Richard J. Murane (Free Press, 1996, $24.00). Drawing on the work of real teachers, parents, and administrators, this book provides a blueprint for turning our schools around.

Things Will Be Different for My Daughter, Mindy Bingham (Penguin Books USA, 1995, $14.95). Handbook to help parents build their daughter's self-esteem throughout each stage of her life by confronting traditional challenges to her success and suggesting ways to overcome them.

What Parents Need to Know About Dating Violence: Learning the Facts and Helping Your Teen, Patricia Occhiuzzo Giggans and Barrie Levy (Seal Press, 1995, $12.95). Defines dating violence, demonstrates the warning signs, and explains the psychology of an abusive relationship and how to help.

The Working Parents Help Book, Susan Crites Price and Tom Price (Peterson's, Princeton, NJ, 1996, $16.95). The classic guide for working parents everywhere. A 1994 *Parents Choice Award* winner (includes windows *Working Parents Helpware* ®).

You and Your Adolescent: A Parent's Guide for Ages 10 to 20, Laurence Steinberg and Ann Levine (HarperCollins, 1990, $19.95) Reassuring

help with the expected and unexpected issues of physical, emotional, and social growth. Highly recommended.

VIOLENCE AND CRIME PREVENTION

1) Acquaintance Rape; 2) What Is Sexual Harassment?; 3) Sexual Harassment; 4) Flirting or Harassment?; and 5) Harassment? Don't Take It!, ETR Associates (P.O. Box 1830, Santa Cruz, CA 95061-1830). For free copies of these five brochures, send a SASE with 75¢ postage. Also available: ***Considering Marriage: Avoiding Marital Violence***, by Lee Bowker.

But What About Me?, Marilyn Reynolds (Morning Glory Press, 6595 San Haraldo Way, Buena Park, CA 90620, 1996, $8.95). Portrays the horrors of acquaintance rape. Written in a "true-to-life" format, the book enlightens without preaching.

Child Lures Family Guide, Kenneth Wooden (Wooden Publishing House, 1996, $4.00; 2119 Shelburne Road, Shelburne, VT 05482; 802-985-8458). Tips for parents for protecting kids from molestation and sexual assault. Endorsed by the American Academy of Pediatrics.

Domestic Violence: What Some Women Live With is a Crime, Aimee Argel (State of Michigan Department of Civil Rights, 1995; 1-800-996-6228; free). Brochure defines domestic violence, the laws, what people can do to stop the cycle of violence.

Don't Be the Next Victim: 50 Ways to Protect Yourself Against Crime, Richard W. Eaves and Steven E. Watson (Guardian Press, 1993, $8.95: 1-800-466-1010). Paperback packed with common-sense, easy-to-follow tips on how to avoid crime.

50 Things You Can Do About Guns, James M. Murray (Robert D. Reed Publishers, 750 La Playa, Suite 647, San Francisco, CA 94121; 1-800-774-7336; $7.95 + $2.50 shipping/-handling). Information to help stop gun violence.

Firearm Facts (Children's Safety Network at the National Center for Education in Maternal and Child Health, 2000 15th Street N., Suite 701, Arlington, VA 22201; 703-524-7802, free). Firearm facts on youth suicide and guns, crime, and preventing injuries.

Crime Prevention Training

Chimera: Self Defense for Women:
312-759-1707 (Chimera Educational Foundation, Inc., 200 N. Michigan, #401, Chicago, IL 60601). Workshops, lectures, and a 12-hour basic self-defense course for women. Offices located in Georgia, Illinois, New Jersey, North Carolina, Ohio, Pennsylvania, and Wisconsin.

Citizens Against Crime: 1-800-466-1010 (P.O. Box 1241, Allen Texas 75002). Crime prevention and personal safety seminars for groups and businesses. Offices located in most major cities.

CRIMEFREE Seminars, Inc.:
313-432-9333 (P.O. Box 2905, Livonia, MI 48150-0905). Presentations on personal crime prevention, child safety, sexual harassment, and home safety. Programs offered in Michigan and northern Ohio.

Keep Your Family Safe from Firearm Injury, the American Academy of Pediatrics and Center to Prevent Handgun Violence (Free: Send SASE legal-size to STOP Brochure, 1225 Eye Street N.W., Suite 1100, Washington, DC 20005; 202-289-7319). Brochure offers tips on how to reduce risks of firearm injury to families.

Kids and Gangs: What Parents and Educators Need to Know, Ann Lawson (Johnson Institute, 7205 Ohms Lane, Minneapolis, MN 55439- 2159; 1-800-231-5165, 1994, $4.95 + 55¢ shipping). A complete picture of gangs: types of gangs, gang behavior, *and* psychological, social, and family dynamics factors that increase the risk of kids joining gangs. This is *not* a book for your teens.

Safe at School: Awareness and Action for Parents of Kids K-12, Carol Silverman Saunders (Free Spirit Publishing Inc., 400 First Avenue N., Suite 616, Minneapolis, MN 55401-1730; 612-338-2068; $14.95 + $4.25 shipping/handling). Helps parents deal with bullying, gangs, sexual harassment, and other safety issues.

Safeguarding Your Children, by The National PTA—The Allstate Foundation (330 N. Wabash Avenue, Suite 2100, Chicago, IL 60611-3690; 312-670-6782, 1995, $4.50 + $3.50 shipping/handling). 30-page booklet full of information on how to help kids deal with all types of danger. Includes excellent resources. Call the National PTA for a complete catalog of booklets and brochures.

1) Stop the Violence: Start Something New; 2) Your Inside Look at Crime Prevention; and *3) Getting Together to Fight Crime: How Working with Others Can Help You Build a Safer and Better Community*, National Crime Prevention Council (Fulfillment Center, P.O. Box 1, 100 Church Street, Amsterdam, NY 12010; 1-800-NCPC-911). Ideas on how parents can help develop successful crime prevention initiatives.

Streetsmarts: A Teenager's Safety Guide, by Jane Goldman (Barron's Educational Series, Inc., 1996, $4.95). Commonsense guide to help teens deal with everyday life: Dating, unwanted sexual advances, coping with bullies, and avoiding unnecessary risks in public places.

Tune in to Your Rights: A Guide for Teenagers About Turning Off Sexual Harassment, Programs for Educational Opportunity (School of Education, University of Michigan, Ann Arbor, MI 48109-1259; 313-763-9910; $4.00). Defines sexual harassment, identifies warning signals, and provides tips for parents and schools.

Voices From The Streets, S. Beth Atkin (Little, Brown and Company, 1996, $17.95). A message of hope, focusing on kids who got out of gangs. Most speak of wishing parents had taking a more active role in their lives.

Help for Domestic Violence
The nationwide **Domestic Violence Hotline:**
1-800-799-7233,   TDD: 1-800-787-3224

Michigan Family Violence hotline:
1-800-996-6228
The Domestic Violence Project SAFE House,
Washtenaw County: 313-995-5444
Domestic Violence Clinic, Wayne County
Legal Services, 9 am-7 pm: 313-962-0466
Common Ground, Pontiac: 810-456-0909
First Step, Westland: 313-459-5900
The Haven, Pontiac: 810-334-1274
Interim House, Detroit: 313-861-5300
LACASA, Livingston Cty: 810-227-7100
My Sister's Place, Detroit: 313-371-3900
Turning Point, Mt. Clemens: 810-463-6990

HELP FOR RUNAWAYS
National Runaway Switchboard:
1-800-621-4000
Covenant House's Nineline: 1-800-999-9999
AT&T and Traveler's Aid Society
of Rhode Island: 1-800-862-3723
Off the Streets (Detroit):   313-824-4520
or 313-873-0678
The Sanctuary (Royal Oak): 810-547-2260

ORDER FORM FOR *HEALTHY TEENS*

Name: _____

Title: _____
Institution/School/
Organization/Business: _____

Address: _____

_____

Phone: (_____) _____ Fax: (_____) _____

NUMBER ORDERED   **PRICE**   **SHIPPING & HANDLING**
   1 to   10 @ $5.95 per copy . . . . $2.00 plus 25¢ per book
  11 to   49 @ $4.50 per copy . . . . $2.00 plus 22¢ per book
  50 to   99 @ $4.00 per copy . . . . 17¢ per book
 100 to   999 @ $3.50 per copy . . . . 13¢ per book
1,000 to 1,999 @ $3.25 per copy . . . . 11¢ per book
2,000 to 2,999 @ $3.00 per copy . . . . 11¢ per book
3,000 to 3,999 @ $2.75 per copy . . . . 11¢ per book
4,000 to 4,999 @ $2.50 per copy . . . . 10¢ per book
5,000 or more @ $2.25 per copy . . . . 10¢ per book

All orders for five or more books are shipped via UPS ground.

QUANTITY _____ X PRICE _____ = _____

Michigan residents add 6% tax: _____

PLUS SHIPPING & HANDLING (see above):   _____

TOTAL AMOUNT: _____

PLEASE MAKE CHECKS PAYABLE TO BRIDGE COMMUNICATIONS, INC.

INSTITUTION BILLING INFORMATION:

[   ] Please invoice our institution, Attn: _____

[   ] Purchase order number: _____
[   ] We will be mailing a purchase order. (Credit extended with purchase
    order.)
[   ] Our tax-exempt ID number is _____

RETURN TO: BRIDGE COMMUNICATIONS, INC., 1450 Pilgrim Road,
Birmingham, MI 48009: FAX: (810) 644-8546
Questions? Feel free to call Marcia (Rayner) Applegate at (810) 646-1020.
E-mail BridgeComm@AOL.com